eat sleep poop

creating balance for wellness

theresa p freeman pt,lmt,chc

Table of Contents

<u>Foreword</u>

When Theresa told me that she was writing a book she would like me to take a look at I was intrigued. I know her to be a bright, well-read health care professional and wellness coach who has taken information and made it her own over the years. I have celebrated with her as she learned the skills of creating health in her own life and caring for her family. I loved reading about her personal journey as well as how she cared for her husband since his cancer diagnosis.

For those of us in the healing professions, it is sometimes difficult to support all the medical and lifestyle choices our family, friends and even clients or patients decide without judging or trying to control them. Theresa navigates this dance with grace and in the process offers insight into honoring the beliefs we each have and reminds us of the importance of meeting people where they are.

When I saw the title of her book, it brought a huge smile to my face. How wonderful to have fun with these cornerstones of our well-being. For, in fact, what else is there but these three little things when it comes to health? *Eat Sleep Poop* is a great resource. This book gets to the guts of what we need to know about how our bodies function and gives practical guidance on how to integrate this knowledge into our lives.

In the past few years more and more books have been written to guide us in nutrition and provide ways to achieve a healthier lifestyle. People are seeking reliable sources of information, and the explosion online and through "Dr. Google" make it both easier to find information and also be overwhelmed by the answers. *Eat Sleep Poop* takes a complicated, interconnected body of knowledge and makes it both understandable and accessible both to health care providers and the general public.

Theresa outlines clearly the relationship between food and health, but this is not just about eating, sleeping and pooping; it is about life.

Susan Ackerly, N.D., C.P.M.
Topsham, Maine

<u>Preface</u>

I used to have this conversation with myself: "If I ever get cancer, I will definitely go vegan or macrobiotic." Then I would laugh at myself with rebuttal: "If that's the healthiest way to eat and prevent or cure illness, then why wait? Just do it *now* and prevent cancer or whatever else might be lurking in my future."

I was first introduced to the vegan-macrobiotic way of eating in my early 30s. It was a great introduction to clean, wholesome and thoughtful eating, but somewhat extreme compared to my Standard American Diet (SAD). I attempted this healthier diet a couple times, but it was difficult to transition to and maintain. It felt rigid and hard to implement in my life as a long-term diet.

While I loved eating clean, whole foods and attending vegan and macrobiotic educational cooking classes, and had even called myself "vegan-ish" in the past, in its pure form this was not an easy lifestyle for me to sustain. My family's diet contained a fair amount of meat and dairy products, so it felt very difficult to make this significant shift to eliminate animal products. It also seemed very foreign to my immediate and extended family. They were not on board which made it even more difficult to fully engage in this lifestyle, even by myself. As a pure diet, it did not work for me. I also found that it fed my "all or nothing" personality, making me more rigid and extreme, and far less fun to be around.

I know this diet works for many people and I admire the lifestyle, but I have learned that for now, I am better with simple, clean eating versus pure vegan-macrobiotic. I continue to dabble in some of the wholesome dishes, eat significantly fewer animal products, and implement many of the healthy eating theories into my life and my health coaching.

We all need to find what's right for us to support a balanced diet and lifestyle to promote our own wellness. As they say in the Institute of Integrative Nutrition (IIN), through which I earned my initial health coaching credentials, it's all about "bio-individuality"—what is right for one person may not be right for another. We each have to create our own personal prescription for wellness.

Recently, my diet and nutrition values were retested and then validated when my husband was diagnosed with a brain tumor. I was a bit overwhelmed thinking about the perfect diet and feeling as if I would need to implement a pure anti-cancer nutrition plan for him and the entire family, immediately. My old way of thinking about the extreme diet change for cancer came rushing in.

I was somewhat perplexed, yet relieved, when the oncology nutritionist told him to simply eat more fruits and vegetables, lean meats and fish, and decrease carbohydrates. Her suggestion was not to do anything extreme. She mentioned the ketogenic diet which I had also learned about while researching brain cancer. This high fat diet has been implemented with some success on some brain cancer patients. But she could tell by my husband's personality, lifestyle and current situation that this was not the time to implement, enforce or encourage such an extremely limiting diet change. She said cancer treatment was not going to be fun and this was not the time to make major changes or feel deprived and make this any harder than it was going to be. She spoke with wisdom and experience, but I did not realize it at the time.

Moving forward, we simply focused on getting through Paul's primary injury, diagnosis, and early treatments without any drastic dietary changes. I continued to cook and serve healthy, balanced meals, but made no major shifts immediately in our menus. We decided to keep our then-basic diet and focused instead on keeping life familiar and simple.

Our nutritionist was right, Paul had been through a lot, and there was still a lot more to come in the cancer process. Initially, he had to recover from a significant concussion, the result of his fall to the pavement on the day he had a seizure caused by his brain tumor. This was followed by brain surgery six days later to remove his small lemon-sized tumor. A month after that, he underwent six intense weeks of combined radiation and chemotherapy. After a month's rest, he endured a year of another 12 cycles of chemotherapy.

On top of this major medical trauma, we were forced to embrace that neither one of us was up for a radical change in diet.

I also realized very quickly that this was primarily *his* cancer journey, not mine, and I did not have the power or ability to control any of it. So, instead, I decided for our greatest success, that I would support him the best I could without forcing any of my extreme ideas on him. We were going to join forces and be a strong team; moving forward together gradually was the master plan.

This cancer journey with my husband has helped me become a much better health coach and life partner. We all are unique with varied needs for optimal health, and all have a vast array of personalities, body types and health and lifestyle requirements. When making changes in diet and lifestyle, a more subtle and gentle approach has led to greater success, both personally and professionally. Instead of imposing my beliefs and judgment, working as a team, collaborating and encouraging has proven best.

A lot of my early health coach training coincided with my husband's acute cancer treatments. As I progressed with classes, I was hearing abundant talk about inflammation, illness and diet. I also began my own research around diet and lifestyle in relation to cancer.

Halfway through Paul's chemotherapy, as we approached the holidays, I felt as if it were time to make some changes. I had let my own healthy diet and lifestyle slip and needed to make some of my own improvements. When the New Year arrived, my husband agreed to pay attention to the foods most known to cause inflammation—sugar and other simple carbohydrates.

He and I had a conversation about how we needed to do our part to minimize inflammation, in order to help prevent the regrowth of cancer. As we neared the end of his chemotherapy and formal medical cancer treatment, we decided to take a more active role in this cancer prevention journey. Prayer was important and profoundly helpful, but we also needed a more palpable approach. I told Paul what I had learned about sugar and simple carbohydrates being the top inflammatory culprits, and how managing these could help decrease the chance of cancer regrowth and even prevent illness and disease.

Paul willingly agreed to make some changes, and we started by decreasing the obvious—white flour and white sugar. He immediately decreased his intake of bread, pasta, crackers, soda and such. Within just one month, we noticed more changes than I had expected. We were both pleased to see that a few subtle adjustments in our diet could lead to some big changes in wellness.

Paul noticed he had more energy, less hunger and fatigue (less "hangry"). He also welcomed the weight loss along with the decreased bloating and puffiness. We both had our validation that to eat well, be well, and feel well, diet and lifestyle changes do not have to be painstaking and extreme. We had our living proof.

Fortunately, my husband has a more moderate personality than my all-or-nothing approach. I quickly came to realize in this situation, for his best success, we had to make smaller changes that would meet his lifestyle and habits. A more subtle shift along with patience and a realistic plan would work best. Thanks to Paul, I learned firsthand that making small doable changes in diet, fostering a healthy lifestyle that is sustainable can also create some very desirable differences in well-being.

Similarly, I often like to reflect on the teachings of one of my favorite saints, Mother Teresa of Calcutta. She led a very serious dedicated life of service and greatness, but professed that it was the small things that she did repeatedly that made her work so profoundly positive. Several quotes attributed to Mother Teresa have inspired both my life and, more recently, my work as a health coach:

> *Doing small things with great love.*
> *I do not agree with the big way of doing things … What matters is the individual.*
> *Be faithful in small things because it is in them that your strength lies.*

I believe in these statements and life lessons and have found them to be true and effective when implemented, even in our attention to diet and lifestyle. Small changes in diet, practiced regularly, can lead to greater success in health and wellness than more radical modifications.

Introduction

Much has already been written about the damage that can be done to the human body by inflammation, as well as the poor eating habits that contribute to the condition. Why, then, yet another book?

As with most authors, I have both personal and professional reasons for wanting to address the topic. My hope is that by doing so I might shed enough light on the subject to help the reader in his or her efforts to avoid inflammation altogether, or at least reduce its impact.

As a helping professional with active practices in physical therapy, massage therapy and health coaching, I have worked in these disciplines for 30 years. I also have a teaching role as an adjunct faculty member in the University of New England's physical therapy graduate program.

I first became aware of inflammation through my role as a physical therapist. My patients were presenting with localized pain, swelling and redness associated with injuries and surgeries. Later, working as a massage therapist, my knowledge of inflammation expanded when clients would admit their frequent use or over-use of caffeine, alcohol and sugar. I often describe these products as *over the counter drugs*, used daily by many people.

More times than I can count I would hear about this typical diet from my clients:

> **Morning**—Multiple cups of coffee on an empty stomach, maybe some orange juice with or without a breakfast of cereal, bread or other baked, simple carbohydrate food, or no food at all.

> **Midday**—More caffeinated beverages, often in the form of soda or sweet tea, after or with lunch, usually consisting of a white bread sandwich.

> **Mid-afternoon**—More caffeine (coffee or soda) to accompany a quick snack from the cupboard, vending machine or convenience store.

> **Evening**—A carbohydrate heavy dinner, often based on (white flour) pasta, along with multiple cocktails or glasses of wine.

This food plan often led to a poor night's sleep, and then the whole pattern would be repeated the next day. Starting the day with coffee to get going, then alcohol at the end of the day to settle down, plus sugar and simple carbohydrates mixed in for quick meals and snacks. This was the norm I often observed.

Some of the obvious effects from this way of eating that I have seen in my office include headaches, muscle tension and overstimulation from the "fight or flight" response, causing slower healing times and delayed responses to treatments. Knowing this, I have focused on bringing more awareness to clients during treatment sessions about the downsides of this diet and lifestyle, encouraging them to create healthier choices. Over time, I continued to become even more convinced of the undeniable connection of inflammation and illness to diet and lifestyle as I trained to become a health and wellness coach.

Besides my professional exposure to the inter-connectedness of diet, wellness and health, my personal experience has also influenced this expansion. This has greatly impacted me and led to my passion and desire to share my knowledge in a book format.

On a more personal level, I suffered from chronic sinus infections in the early 1990s. Beginning each fall and continuing into spring, I inevitably contracted numerous colds that would morph into sinus infections that often required antibiotics. Eventually, my forward-thinking OB-Gyn doctor, who knew there was a better path to wellness than taking antibiotics on a regular basis, referred me to a terrific naturopathic doctor, who quickly became an integral part of my personal health care team.

She started by educating me about food sensitivities and mucous-producing foods. She strongly encouraged that I try an elimination diet for six-plus weeks. I hesitantly agreed and focused on abstaining from foods that contained wheat, sugar and dairy, or "wheat, sweet and dairy" as I often call this problematic trio. The choices I deleted were primarily foods that contained white flour, white sugar, and milk along with other dairy products.

The difference this change made in my sinus issues was remarkable, even eye-opening. I was quickly impressed by how much better I felt without these foods in my diet. From that point on, my awareness and excitement around nutrition and its direct effect on my health grew. I began attending vegan and macrobiotic cooking classes offered by local and nationally known natural food enthusiasts. I was rolling my own sushi, making miso soup, stuffing giant squash and baking yummy vegan and gluten free chocolate cakes. I even dabbled in green drinks that I was not too sure about at the time.

Over time, through personal experience and with more information from my naturopath, I learned of many more connections between my food choices and my health status.

EATING TOO MUCH OF THIS ...	... OFTEN LED TO THIS
Simple carbohydrates, caffeine	Stress, anxiety, sleep disturbances
Caffeine, alcohol, sugar	Sleep disturbances; bladder, mood and energy problems
Caffeine	Muscle tension, e.g. neck and jaw tightness
Tomato products, sugar, alcohol	Canker sores, rosacea-type symptoms and/or cold sores
Dairy, milk-based sweets (primarily ice cream and yogurts); white flour foods (pasta, breads, baked goods, etc.)	Sinus issues, congestions, headaches, bowel changes
Fiber, red meat, and/or simple carbohydrates	Gas, bloating, indigestion, "gut ache"
Simple carbohydrates	Fluctuating blood sugar levels leading to excessive hunger, fatigue, irritability

I used to be dependent on caffeine and sugar for afternoon energy. I would drink Diet Coke with lunch then eat cookies and chocolate or treats in the afternoon along with more coffee or strong caffeinated tea. I had mood and energy swings that seemed to be related to low blood sugar which in turn left me tired and hungry. My highs and lows were directly related to my diet and lifestyle, and were caused by fluctuations in my blood sugar levels. I also learned that white flour behaved in my body just like white sugar. Cakes, cookies, pasta, bread, crackers, etc. are all similar once they enter the stomach.

During the year, my summer ice cream and fruity drinks rolled into Halloween candy which turned into Thanksgiving pies that floated into Christmas cookies, homemade fudge and eggnog. (I have a headache just thinking about eating these.)

Fortunately the New Year came with the opportunity to start anew. If by mid-February I had not cleaned up my food, I would vow to begin again with Lent and abstain from all those pesky treats for 40 days. But then I would often have to start all over again after indulging with jelly beans and chocolate bunnies at Easter.

When I over-indulged in certain items (whether in a single episode or from a cumulative effect over a period of time), I would often notice a certain set of symptoms developing. When I tuned in and eliminated or altered consumption of a certain product, the symptoms would usually subside. As I improved my diet, the effects of food became much clearer. Over the course of time, I have become significantly more body-aware. It is obvious that my food and drink habits have a direct effect on my mental and physical well-being.

Through the years, as my passion for and interest in nutrition grew, I easily adopted the truth that *food is medicine.* I learned about the powers of food, both for the betterment and detriment of my health. I began to feel like a living science experiment, and I still do. Usually, when I have an imbalance in the body-mind, I reflect on my diet. More often than not, I find an association or relationship between the two.

I continue to be a strong believer that food can be a curse or a cure. With what I am eating, I could be feeding the fire when I should be putting it out. A poor diet can cause illness and imbalances in the body and mind. In turn, it is clear that a properly balanced diet can promote optimal health and wellness. Making small dietary changes and eating better has the ability to alter or impact health in a positive way. This has been proven many times both at home and work.

Although I do not have a perfect diet, I eat with an increased awareness around the powers of food. I have learned through studying and personal experience that the 90:10 rule can be very effective. My diet is healthy most of the time

(90%), but not all the time. Ten percent of the time, I allow myself some of the items that are not optimal for a clean, balanced diet. I still eat wheat-sweet-dairy, but in moderation. I also partake in modest amounts of caffeine, alcohol and sugar, but attempt to respect their potential drug-like effects.

There are times when I violate my 90:10 rule, usually during holidays with traditional desserts and celebratory treats and drinks, or during the summer months with trips to the ice cream store and my favorite seasonal drink of sangria. My motto remains, however, "It's what we do most of the time, not some of the time." It is OK to have a little cake to celebrate a birthday, but maybe not for *every* office birthday event. Similarly, it's OK to be social and gather with friends and family for a drink, but not *multiple* drinks at each event. It's important to learn how to say, "No thank you," and implement other healthy options.

I clearly notice that if I deviate from my food boundaries for too long, my health suffers and my body speaks to me. Sometimes this sensitivity is bothersome and annoying, but I am grateful for the awareness and messages my body gives me. I have come to see this as a blessing rather than a burden. All in all, my body keeps me honest and unable to step out of line for very long. I will often experience headaches, insufficient sleep, sinus congestion, energy or mood swings, anxiousness and brain fog. I notice that I have become quite sensitive with a heightened awareness around how foods make me feel. When I am not feeling well or just feeling a bit off, food is usually the first thing I look at. What am I eating a lot of that is not beneficial for my health? Or, what am I *not* eating? What's missing?

I have been amazed at how biological and innate the process of wellness can be. For example, I have now expanded my awareness to include my sleep and exercise. I often monitor myself and ask, "What is the quality of my sleep? Do I need more? Am I getting enough exercise? Do I need more upbeat (cardio) workouts or something more gentle, such as yoga or long walks? Do I need to increase my strength training?"

Often it will occur to me that what I need most is to relax, rather than do more, more, more, since adrenaline can be a drug too. As awareness expands, I might find myself asking, "How much fresh air am I getting? Where is my spirituality? Are my relationships in order? How is my balance between work and play, being busy and having down time?" In The Institute of Integrated Nutrition, these other areas are referred to as "primary foods" and have a very important place in wellness along with edible food.

Continuing in reference to food, small amounts of caffeine, alcohol, sugar, and carbohydrates are not always bad, but it is important for them not to consume and take over our health. If eating them in moderation does not work, then maybe eliminating them from our diet will be necessary. Sometimes I need to clean up my diet and push the reset button, then resettle into the 90:10 rule. The 90:10 rule is what I practice most of the time. That's where I feel best. Over the years, it has worked best for me and many of my clients, but it does not work all the time for everyone. Extreme or perfect diets can lead to rigid lifestyles and feed the troubling perfectionist personality and be socially limiting.

I have learned that some of my clients, those for whom the 90:10 rule does not work, may be suffering from food *addiction*. For these people, abstinence from certain foods is best. Just as alcoholics can not take that first drink, these food addicts cannot just have one cookie or dessert, occasional wine or coffee, for example, or just a little of whatever triggers the addiction and leads to a binge. My best recommendation for this situation is to consult with a trusted doctor or investigate a support group, such as one of the food-related Twelve-Step programs, e.g. Food Addicts Anonymous or Overeaters Anonymous.

In addition to fostering an addiction, certain foods can cause a full range of sensitivities or allergic reactions. In fact, small amounts of certain foods such as peanuts or shellfish can trigger a full-blown fatal reaction in some people. Another issue is gluten sensitivity, and those with this or, more seriously, celiac disease may experience digestive distress (gas, bloating, pain) that accumulates and worsens over time.

The symptoms to look for that may be pointing to a food-related illness—some of which I have experienced myself—include headache, red or watery eyes, eyelid styes, nasal congestion, irritability, a frequent sense of extreme hunger, food cravings, fatigue, muscle aches, canker sores, cold sores, rashes, acne, sleep disturbances, swelling of the hands or feet, changes in bowel and bladder patterns (urgency, frequency, constipation or loose stools), bloating and gassiness.

All of these symptoms are keys to understanding inflammation, and I have narrowed the most influential and troublesome areas to three: sugar, sleep and digestion. (Or, in simpler terms, "Eat, Sleep and Poop.") As a mother, this makes sense since one of the more practical ways to measure the wellness of my children has been to look for how they are eating, sleeping and pooping. The concept works just as well with adults, especially my clients. If these three basic daily activities are in order, then they feel better, more balanced and well.

I am not a purist or a perfectionist, nor do I advocate for any particular diet, but I *have* learned how to manage my health with respect to food and lifestyle. I am eager to share some of the things I have learned, both personally and professionally. My hope is to continue helping others better manage their health too.

<u>MEDICAL DISCLAIMER</u>

The information in this book is to be considered complementary to, rather than a replacement for, treatment by trained health care professionals. It is not meant to take the place of any necessary medical care or management of serious illness, but is offered to supplement and possibly prevent the onset or advancement of inflammatory disease. Working with a doctor or specialized nutritionist may be essential. Basic knowledge can be helpful in maintaining health and preventing excess inflammation that can lead to illness and disease. Education, along with practicing a good healthy lifestyle is of utmost importance to help prevent disease and to complement health care.

Please be sure to seek medical attention for any signs or symptoms of significant or lasting illness.

<u>Chapter 1: Inflammation</u>

Inflammation can be our friend and our enemy. It is a natural and necessary response in our body that promotes healing and maintains balance and order. In excess, it can interfere with natural immune system and cell functions, leading to organ damage, illness and disease.

We have all heard the saying, *"You can't live with it and you can't live without it."* Maybe this sounds like some other more personal and familiar relationship? Not unlike human relationships, this is one we cannot go without and needs to be nurtured or it can become volatile.

William Meggs, M.D., Ph.D., and Carol Svec, M.A., said it perfectly when they wrote in their 2004 book *The Inflammation Cure* that it's all about "balancing pro-inflammatory versus anti-inflammatory."

It is important to help minimize the underlying excessive inflammatory process rather than "feed it." As we progress through this book, I will help make sense of inflammation and how it relates to us as individuals in our daily habits and what we can do to better manage it. We will start by gaining a better understanding of what inflammation is.

I love the term *inflammaging*. This is a term coined by researchers from the Norwich Research Park in the U.K. They define it as "low-grade inflammation that increases with age"—perfectly described in a nutshell for us.

Over time, with age, our bodies naturally have an increase in inflammation leading to a variety of diseases and illnesses. We can either fuel this cycle of breaking down cells and taxing our system with extra work or we can promote healthy cells and tissues while supporting our organ functions. With some conscious effort, we can help manage the excess trouble by developing healthy habits. Aging is a naturally occurring biological process that we seem to have a limited degree of power and control over. In actuality, there are many simple and very doable things we can do within our diet and lifestyle to help manage the speed of our body's degradation and improve the quality of our health.

How can we tell if we are living with excess inflammation in our body? There are a number of ways.

There are numerous medical tests that can be used, but to be effective the level of inflammation needs to be advanced enough to be detectable. Ideally, we would like to prevent reaching these levels.

Some of these procedures include the following:

A simple blood test, **CBC or complete blood count**, can detect a rise in white blood cells (WBC). This is often a basic measure of inflammation marked by certain cells increasing to fight a possible infection or inflammation process in the body.

One of the most relevant inflammation markers is **C-reactive protein**, better known as CRP. This can be measured in the blood and is a protein synthesized by the liver. This shows a general level of inflammation existing in the body without specificity to location. CRP is often used as a starting point or an early diagnostic tool. An elevated level may suggest an infection or chronic long-term disease process occurring. This may be a precursor to further testing as well as a follow up assessment tool. It is often utilized in the midst of treatment to assess and reassess for changes, hopefully for improvements over time.

Hyperinsulinism is another inflammatory marker. An excess of sugar and carbohydrates in the diet can lead to elevated blood sugar, causing hyperinsulinism. Increased blood sugar (BS) and insulin levels can be detected in the blood. One of the obvious diseases associated with these increased levels is diabetes or even pre-diabetes.

Hemoglobin A1C (HbA1c) is a blood test measuring glucose and is most often used to help diagnose diabetes as well as measuring diabetic blood sugar management. In basic terms, this is a blood test measure of the average glucose levels over a period of three months. At certain levels, this would indicate inflammation in the body in relation to blood sugar. This can also relate to brain function and has a direct correlation to memory. In my recent functional medicine training, Dee Harris and Dr. David Perlmutter, MD cite studies that show levels of HbA1c above 5.2 indicate decreased memory and a smaller size of the hippocampus, which is where the memory center is located in the brain. In the October 2013, Journal of Neurology by Winkler, et al, the primary study was "Higher glucose levels associated with lower memory and reduced hippocampal microstructure.".

With a rise in blood sugar, there is often a concurrent rise in **cytokines**. Cytokines are small protein cells that communicate with other cells to stimulate and help manage the immune or inflammatory response. Different types of cytokines are released by the immune system and communicate with various cells to either increase or decrease the inflammatory response in the body. This can be measured in the blood and can give specific information as to where the inflammation is and what disease process it may be related to. For example, high levels of a particular cytokine such as interferon or interleukin have been associated with:

- anxiety
- hypertension
- cardiovascular risk
- certain cancers
- Alzheimer's
- rheumatoid arthritis

Advanced inflammation shows up in a variety of well-known diseases, including but not limited to:

- Alzheimer's
- arthritis, asthma
- auto-immune diseases
- cancer
- coronary artery disease
- depression
- diabetes
- irritable bowel syndrome (IBS)

In the early phase of a disease, before it becomes full-blown and detectable by medical testing, there is often a low level of smoldering inflammation. This could be occurring for years and have long-term effects, leading to disease and illness. There may or may not be symptoms coinciding with this lingering low level inflammatory process.

Prevention is truly the best treatment for illness and disease. Whether there is currently an illness or disease process brewing, it is always better to adopt new habits of health in diet and lifestyle rather than wait for something to show up on a medical test.

Prevention of major illness and medical intervention is key. To spend less time and money on doctors' appointments, medical tests and treatments, medications and procedures can make a huge difference in life. Experiencing less physical pain, along with the mental and emotional stress of being sick is the biggest reward.

Herein lies a major reason to promote the anti-inflammatory diet and lifestyle sooner rather than later, and to prevent a full-blown disease process, whether or not signs and symptoms are present.

Early in the inflammatory process, our body may be presenting subtle hints of ill health brewing. If we listen and make some changes, we may be able to prevent acceleration and even reverse symptoms.

These are some low level, early warning inflammatory signs and can be very helpful if we pay attention. They will vary in location and intensity depending on the cause and relevant body system.

A starter or partial list may include:

* aches in joints or muscles
* bloating
* bowel or bladder symptoms
* congestion
* fatigue
* headaches
* mood disorders
* sleep disturbances
* puffy or red irritated eyes
* skin rashes or redness

Maybe these signs have been experienced today or in the past week, month or year? Might they be related to poor dietary habits, stress or lack of exercise and purposeful activity?

Many of these symptoms can often be improved or managed with a few healthy diet or lifestyle changes. Too often they advance, requiring more significant medical attention. By taking some early actions, we can save unnecessary losses of time, money and energy.

Excess inflammation in the body is truly the root of most evil doings with regard to illness. Medical evidence continues to show that the majority of disease is caused by excess inflammation in the body and can be preventable with improved habits in our diet and lifestyle.

Is it truly possible to control or change the course of our health? Many people believe that health is predetermined by their family medical history. They may have a predisposition toward certain genetic tendencies, but this does *not* confirm a doomed destiny for certain illnesses.

Certainly, there is a correlation between illness and disease with regard to genetics, but it is not the sole determinant. Nutrition and behaviors play a huge role in the manifestation of these diseases, and we can make personal choices to significantly influence their occurrence.

We can apply this to a similar theory: *nature versus nurture* or *biological versus behavioral.*

We are all born with a particular genetic makeup from our parents and ancestors, but we can enhance or diminish the outcomes by our behavior and how we live our lives. For example, an astounding fact is that less than five percent of cancers are genetically inherited. This means that 95 percent are caused by lifestyle, or what we are either exposed to or ingest.

As reported by the non-profit organization Cancer Research UK in June 2015, "Genetic specialists estimate that only about 2 or 3 in every 100 cancers diagnosed (2 to 3 percent) are linked to an inherited gene fault." They add that it usually takes six or more gene faults before cancer develops.

Cancers that are not caused by inherited genetic mutations can sometimes appear to "run in families." For example, a shared environment or lifestyle, such as tobacco use, can cause similar cancers to develop among family members.

"Even if a cancer-predisposing mutation is present in a family, not everyone who inherits the mutation will necessarily develop cancer. Several factors influence the outcome," according to an April 2015 report from the National Cancer Institute. They advise genetic counseling to help sort out the risk factors for developing cancer.

The chances of repeating a family history of illness are much greater if we eat the same foods and live the same lifestyles as our parents, extended family members or ancestors. But, if healthy habits are developed, these chances of repeating an unhealthy family medical history are significantly decreased or diminished. In many cases, we have the power to turn genes on or off by the choices we make in diet and lifestyle and what we may or may not be exposed to in our environment. The term for this is epigenetics, which references the ability of genes to be switched on or off. It is very exciting to be immersed in this information regarding diet and lifestyle influencing genetic expression.

A few common preventable ailments are obesity, adult onset diabetes and heart disease. Other disease processes that can be short circuited include many cancers and autoimmune diseases. This may seem like a bold statement, but it has been proven repeatedly in research. I have also heard numerous people tell of their improvements, recovery and prevention from what was thought to be a "family disease." I also have seen numerous clients experience remarkable positive changes in medical testing by improving their diet and lifestyle. One recent case was a health coach client who had a non-alcohol related liver disease. After making significant improvements in lifestyle, this person saw notable improvements in liver enzyme levels (50 percent improvement), substantial weight loss and increased energy.

Moving forward, we will focus on a few very doable and effective ways to help decrease inflammation, improve our current health and help prevent future health issues. By understanding the "why and how" of inflammation, we will become more educated, take greater initiative and become more motivated to achieve optimal health for getting well and staying well.

"An ounce of prevention is worth a pound of cure."
-Benjamin Franklin-

Chapter 2: Sugar & Glycemic Index (GI)

When it comes to inflammation, sugar is probably the number one fuel that feeds the fire.

This book could start and end right here. If we could eliminate all sugar and its equivalents, we would stomp out more sickness than imaginable.

One of my favorite quotes from a dear client, "Sugar is party food for inflammation." She understands this concept all too well as she is currently living with multiple sclerosis (MS), an autoimmune disease that some studies have shown benefits from an anti-inflammatory diet.

Sugar is considered to be one of the world's worst culprits in our diets, with harmful effects including life-changing diseases and illness. This is most often related to the resulting inflammation. Sugar is sugar is sugar, but there are many more foods that mimic sugar in our diets and that can be extremely detrimental to our health. To better understand this, it is important to learn about glucose in the body and what is known as the *glycemic index* (GI).

Glucose is the number one energy source for the body. It derives primarily from carbohydrates in our diet. When we eat actual sugar or simple carbohydrates, they convert to glucose in our bodies. A certain amount is essential for us to function, but in excess it causes trouble in the form of inflammation, fat and bodily dysfunction.

Other sources of fuel for our body are protein and fat which are *not* immediately converted into glucose and do not have the direct effect on blood glucose that carbohydrates do. As a matter of fact, in conjunction with fiber, fat can actually help slow digestion and absorption, aiding in the balance of blood sugar. When attention is given to the quality of protein and fat, these macronutrients can be very beneficial in minimizing inflammation.

Carbohydrates and glucose demand a release of insulin from the pancreas to turn food into fuel for the body to use. Through the colon, glucose and insulin enter the bloodstream and travel to various organs and muscles. Insulin turns most of the extra glucose to glycogen which is then stored in muscles and the liver for energy to be used at a later time. If too much glucose is produced, it is released in the blood for recirculation or excretion. In excess, it is also stored as fat. Organ fat versus subcutaneous fat is the most detrimental. Two of the most harmful fat stores are belly fat and liver fat.

Over time, higher glucose levels in the body can cause an overloading demand on the pancreas for insulin and cause a decrease in insulin sensitivity. With decreased efficiency, glucose cannot be properly converted to energy and causes a detrimental excess in the body. This can become a vicious cycle. With decreased insulin sensitivity, there will be higher blood sugar levels. This excess glucose can cause increased body fat and inflammation, and lead to or cause illnesses such as diabetes and heart disease.

Weight gained from extra body fat can also decrease insulin effectiveness. If insulin is ineffective, then there will be increased glucose circulating in the blood. Increased blood sugar levels lead to increased inflammation, disease and illness. And on and on it goes. Increased glucose demands increased insulin and decreases insulin sensitivity which increases glucose levels which causes increased fat, which decreases insulin effectiveness, and again, increases glucose. As previously stated, this vicious cycle creates a breeding ground for inflammation, illness and disease.

Most healthy bodies are very efficient and can easily manage fluctuating glucose levels by releasing more insulin. But if we chronically abuse this system over time, our bodies can be overtaxed and wear out, losing the ability to manage efficiently. This in turn can cause inflammation and compromised health. As earlier listed, diabetes, heart disease, cancers and Alzheimer's are just a few of the possible resulting issues.

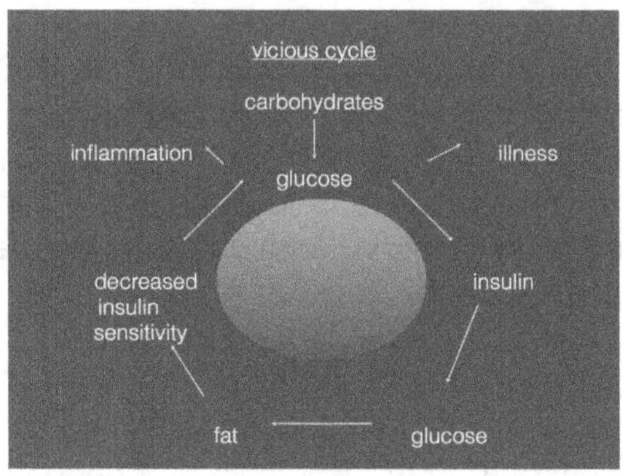

To be more preventive, it is important to learn how to affect blood sugar and thus better manage excess inflammation. In order to do that, it is necessary to learn about the importance of the glycemic index mentioned above and developed at the University of Toronto in 1981.

Glycemic index, in short, is a value placed on a food based on how that food affects the glucose or blood sugar levels in the body.

The place to look to begin understanding GI is carbohydrates, as they have a close but not exact association with this index. A familiar nutrient that we can actually measure, carbohydrates are usually calculated in grams. It is relatively easy to determine the quantity of carbohydrates in a food by reading labels, or if necessary, referring to books, Internet sources or even some smartphone applications. This is a great place to start, to become more aware of our carbohydrate intake, which is oftentimes excessive. But simply knowing and minimizing our carbohydrate consumption is not enough to optimize health and minimize inflammation. We also need to evaluate the quality of low or non-carbohydrate foods we eat and to understand the variety and value of the other carbohydrates we ingest.

Not all carbs are created equal. The quick explanation to that statement is that carbohydrates can be categorized into *simple* (quickly absorbed) or *complex* (slowly absorbed). This distinction is not typically broken down for us on food packaging and labels. Usually, we just know if something generally contains carbohydrates. Understanding GI can help us better differentiate between the quality of foods based on how they affect our glucose levels.

GI ratings can be found in books, online or even on some nutritional labels and are based on a scale of 0-100.

- Low GI foods are rated 0-55 (oatmeal is 53)
- Medium GI foods are rated 56-69 (white bread is 69)
- High GI foods are rated 70-100 (pure glucose is 100)

Once we start to learn more about the categories and differences in the GI of foods, we will see that an actual number rating or chart is not necessary to understand the system and still be successful. Personally, I rarely utilize the formal number charts. I rely on the basic understanding of *low versus high* to better balance my diet and combine certain foods to help maintain balanced blood sugar levels and promote wellness.

Food pairings is a term I like to use in reference to GI. This may be familiar in other situations like wine and food pairings. I choose to apply it here in the sense of food combinations to help manage blood sugar levels. My goal is to teach others to utilize similar thinking.

A few quick and rough not-so-healthy examples include topping ice cream and hot fudge with nuts; eating cheese and whole grain crackers with wine; or having peanuts with beer. Healthier examples include adding high-quality lean protein and fat (e.g. cheese, chicken, fish, eggs, seeds, nuts) to a salad; using peanut butter on a whole-grain English muffin or toast instead of butter and pairing these with orange juice; or eating a handful of nuts with a fruit or fruit juice.

Speaking anecdotally, my grandmother used to eat a slice of cheese with her apple pie and, as we know, Grammy knows best. She lived to be 101 and I can still hear her say, *"Apple pie without cheese is like a kiss without a squeeze."*

Put simply, the goal here is to increase fat and protein to decrease the glycemic index. We will delve into this in the next chapter where we will learn more about balancing the glycemic index to decrease inflammation. For now, to better understand which foods to combine it is helpful to look more closely at the different *levels* of glycemic index.

Low Glycemic Index. It is easiest to remember that *low is slow.* These foods are more slowly digested and absorbed. In everyday life, this is the most favorable. These minimize the draw on insulin and help prevent extreme sugar highs and lows with fewer spikes in blood sugar levels. Insulin and glucose levels are more easily maintained with lower glycemic foods. Low GI foods allow for a slower release of glucose and insulin, which helps to minimize inflammation in the body.

Low GI foods also give a more satiated feeling. They can be helpful in minimizing excess hunger and lessening frequent cravings. In turn, these help with weight control and maintenance of a more moderate and healthy food intake.

Many low GI foods are often referred to as *complex carbohydrates*. Grains are a good example, especially the less refined ones like slow cooking oats and brown rice. Whole foods and foods with fiber tend to be of lower GI and are considered to be complex carbohydrates. (The term *whole foods* is used frequently, but may not be well understood. These are foods that are grown, not manufactured, and are usually eaten in totality rather than peeled, processed or overly refined.)

Typically, glycemic index is used to categorize carbohydrate-type foods, but in the following examples, I am including proteins and fats. This information can aid in better understanding the general idea of applying GI to our everyday lives, to make sense of certain foods and their effects on blood sugar, and to learn how to integrate the better quality foods and proper combinations in our diets.

With my own personal twist on glycemic index, I will, therefore, place most high protein and fat-based foods in the low GI category. They have very little effect on blood sugar and can actually help balance higher GI foods when eaten together.

Examples of low glycemic foods include:

- Animal proteins such as fish, chicken, beef, pork, shellfish and eggs
- Nuts and seeds (healthy fats rich in monounsaturated fats and omega-3s)
- Tofu and beans (black, red, kidney and garbanzo)

- Vegetables such as broccoli, kale, seaweed, asparagus and cauliflower
- Grains, including brown rice, quinoa, barley, buckwheat and oats
- Oils and fats (olive and canola oil, butter and the fruit avocado, often used as a fat)

Within this group, there is a whole spectrum of quality that needs attention to ensure that choices represent the highest degree of healthiness, or what I consider to be "clean products." These considerations include whether a food is organic, locally grown or factory produced, or genetically modified (GMO). Also important is thinking about lean proteins and quality fats as being better than fat-laden proteins or healthy versus unhealthy fats.

For example, wild-caught rather than farm-raised fishes are considered healthier since the latter often contain more toxins by virtue of being raised in crowded and stressful living spaces, and from swimming in and ingesting their own waste. Similarly, organic, locally raised, grass- or grain-fed meats (chicken, pork and beef) are better for us than those from factory farmed industrialized animals that have been raised in cages and given excessive amounts of antibiotics and hormones.

Medium Glycemic Index. Foods in this category include sweet potatoes, corn, millet, squash, carrots, apples, pears and popcorn. Some of these foods (carrots and apples) will vary in GI depending on how they are prepared. For example, raw fruits and vegetables have a lower glycemic index than those cooked, and the longer these foods are cooked the higher their GI rating will be. In addition, fruits and vegetables eaten with skin on (apples, pears, potatoes) contain more fiber and have lower GI ratings.

Riper fruits have a higher glycemic index and are processed more quickly, spiking blood sugar levels (think a banana with brown rather than yellow skin). The most prevalent genetically modified (GMO) foods to think about include corn, popcorn and soy.

High Glycemic Index. To complete our understanding of GI, it is important to take a look at high GI foods. Unlike the *low is slow* of low GI items, *high is fast* (without the rhyme) is the key here as these choices are those that are most quickly digested. This is the grouping of foods to be more avoided and cautious when considering.

Also considered to be high carbohydrate foods, these foods are rapidly transformed into glucose, causing a quick release of insulin. This extra insulin not only causes an inflammatory response but also leads to increased hunger sooner. The earlier response with cravings for more food is usually for more quick carbohydrates or as we say, *carbs crave carbs*. An increased insulin drive occurs, causing the need for more glucose or carbohydrate type foods. I refer to many of these foods as being nutritionally *empty*. When eating a lot of these foods, especially alone, the body responds as if it never received proper nutrition and leads it to want more.

Physiologically, this change in insulin and glucose actually leads to an increase in the hunger hormone called *ghrelin* and a decrease in the satiation hormone *leptin*.

The body knows that it did not get proper nourishing food and sends the message to eat more in hopes of obtaining more nutrient dense foods. The body's natural response is a desire for proper nourishment to help the body function properly to maintain wellness.

Many high GI foods are high in starch or sugars and are often known as *simple carbohydrates.* Refined and processed foods tend to be of higher GI. If eaten in excess, they often lead to weight gain as well as feeding the inflammatory process.

Examples of high glycemic foods include white potatoes, white rice, and foods with the primary ingredients of white flour and white sugar (e.g., breads, pasta, muffins and cookies, pies, doughnuts and other baked goods). This list also includes alcohol, potato chips, and even bananas and orange juice.

While coffee and caffeine are not typically included among high GI foods, I like to include them because they can have the same effects as a high GI food.

There is also a wide spectrum of quality and GI range to consider within this group. For example, a banana does not have a GI as high or as bad as a piece of fudge, and a whole orange has a lower GI than refined orange juice. Even pure cane sugar and other sweeteners can be prioritized, with dark molasses and pure maple syrup measuring lower on the GI scale than high fructose corn syrup and refined white table sugar.

Some of these high GI foods are often used on a daily basis and can have detrimental health repercussions over time. Many of us add white sugar to our daily coffee or tea and even to breakfast cereals.

I can still remember eating Rice Krispies or puffed rice cereal with low-fat milk and white sugar sprinkled on top for breakfast. I was usually hungry in a short period of time, craving something quick and yummy. Eating a small bowl of whole grain cereal with nuts and fruit would be a much better balanced breakfast and certainly more satisfying.

As mentioned earlier, my husband made some anti-inflammatory diet changes to help manage cancer progression and prevention. He has been practicing a more balanced carbohydrate, glycemic index type diet, not fully eliminating carbohydrates, but balancing and decreasing them. Paul started eating more low GI type foods like high quality mixed nuts for snacks along with fruit and fewer high GI foods like white, refined foods such as white pasta, potatoes, bread and rice.

It has been empowering to have a sense of taking back his own health along with the innumerable added benefits including weight loss and increased energy. Outside of a little shopping for some new clothes and a few extra tailoring fees, it has been a small price to pay for increased wellness.

<u>Chapter 3: Managing This *Sweet* Info</u>

The goal is to control blood sugar levels and slow the rate of digestion in order to improve health by minimizing inflammation and managing appetite and weight.

This will help decrease the dramatic, continuous spikes and drops in glucose and insulin. This also will help minimize the stress and extra workload on the pancreas, which releases insulin, and help maintain its efficiency.

It is important to recognize that "not all foods are created equal." Wellness is not simply about counting calories to promote health and managing weight. Knowing how many calories are in foods can be helpful along with portion control, but much more important is the *quality* of the foods we eat. Fortunately, some of the popular diet programs are starting to consider this.

Thinking about food quality is crucial to overall health and the prevention of illness. Many people continue to think good health is simply controlling weight by balancing calories. "Calories in, calories out," or in other words, eating what we want and exercising enough to burn excess calories. We know through science that there is more to health and preventing illness and disease. Maintaining a proper weight is only part of the health equation.

To promote health, we need to maintain a healthy weight, but we also need to learn to control excess inflammation. One of the primary ways to achieve this is by paying attention to our intake of sugar and carbohydrates and the concomitant effect on glucose levels.

Developing sustainable healthy diet and lifestyle habits, rather than yo-yo dieting, can more effectively lead to ongoing wellness and weight management. Many people lose weight while dieting, then gain most, if not all and more weight back when they return to their old ways. Habits that can be developed and maintained over a lifetime rather than just for a brief period of time are the most effective. Rather than a brief extreme diet change to lose weight for a special occasion, e.g. a wedding or a class reunion, it is more desirable and healthier for long-term lifestyle habits to make lifelong sustainable changes.

In my recent Functional Medicine Coaching Academy training, I learned about *food plans* instead of diets, which gives a better sense of longterm lifestyle changes instead of brief diets without lasting results.

How do we do this?

The ultimate way to begin is to develop a plan to choose one or two simple habits to alter for a week or two, then reassess and tweak or adopt a new simple healthy habit and practice that for a few more weeks. Again, review what is happening both mentally and physically then repeat this process over and over again, continually being aware of the subtle, or not so subtle effects on health and wellness. Healthy habits beget healthy habits, the same way that poor choices create more poor choices leading to perpetual poor health.

Oftentimes, a few small, subtle shifts can lead to bigger and healthier lifestyle changes. The healthier we become, the healthier we want to be. Choices of wellness create continued choices in wellness. For example, if we drink soda on a daily basis, we may decide to try seltzer water with a splash of citrus instead. In turn, we may find ourselves making other healthy choices such as salad or soup with vegetables and lean protein instead of burgers and fries. We may even feel inspired to go for a walk during lunch or after work.

After just small improvements, our personal awareness becomes heightened as we practice healthier behaviors. We tend to notice more how we feel based on our foods, drinks and activities, or lack of.

Each healthy choice we make can bring us a feeling of accomplishment and a desire for more. We continue to string together little victories and start to feel pride and success bringing us to even more positive results.

The more we make healthy choices, the less inclined we are to make unhealthy choices. There is a phrase in health and diet circles called "crowding out." This means focusing on adding quality to diet and lifestyle rather than concentrating only on eliminating poor health habits. Simple examples include adding another vegetable to our plate and opting for salad or soup instead of bread or a heavy appetizer. Both of these choices leave us with less room on the plate, in our stomachs, or in our lives and schedules for the less healthy options.

By focusing on the add-ins instead of the takeaways, we feel less deprived and more inspired, both mentally and physically.

Little by little, we can initiate healthy changes and additions and watch the unhealthy foods and habits fade on their own. By implementing small ways of achieving wellness, we feel more inspired to adopt more healthy behaviors and let go of the not so healthy ones.

One suggestion is to read through the following habits to see which are appealing, then follow your natural instincts. Choose something very doable and not overly daunting. Keep it simple. Implement the lifestyle change for a week or two and see how it feels. Decide if it is time to try something new or to do more of the same. Maybe the alteration feels right and it's time to add another healthy habit. Give it a try!

Here are a few good suggestions to get started on the road to healthy eating:

*Choose **low glycemic** foods.* Focus on quality lean proteins, healthy fats and fiber rich foods. These are usually the complex versus simple carbohydrates. These will help slow digestion and absorption, promoting decreased hunger and less inflammation.

What makes a quality **protein**? Whether it be an animal product or a plant-based product, it is one that occurs with minimal processing and is grown in its most natural form, free of chemicals, artificial ingredients, growth hormones and antibiotics. These would include organic nuts, tofu, chicken, pork, beef, turkey, and wild rather than farm-raised fish and seafood.

What is a healthy **fat**? Typically it is best to eat more plant-based (olive, coconut, avocado) oils and fats rather than animal-based. (The one exception is that which comes from fresh, wild fish.) All of these choices contain essential omega-3 fatty acids.

And what are **fiber** rich foods? Often these are whole fruits and vegetables, nuts and seeds and whole grains. Animal products have little to no fiber. Even though these foods are of a lower glycemic index, by themselves, or in excess, they can be detrimental to our health. People who eat a great deal of meat, chicken and dairy products ingest less fiber and are more prone to colon and gastrointestinal issues including colon cancer and inflammatory bowel disease (IBD) as well as insulin and glucose issues.

*Eat more **whole foods** and **minimally processed** foods.* This means avoiding refined, overly processed, prepackaged and "store bought" foods. I like the phrase I learned in health coach training, *"plants versus plants."* This means focusing on eating plants that are grown instead of foods that come from manufacturing plants. These "real" foods tend to be more nutrient-dense and are easier for the body to digest and utilize, leading to a more satiated feeling while leaving our bodies more satisfied and less hungry. And, these items tend to have lower glycemic indices.

*Eat and cook with more **complex whole grains**.* Explore the various options for pastas, breads and flours. The variety of these continues to expand with new flour-based products being introduced all the time, e.g. whole wheat, brown rice, oat, almond, coconut, and even garbanzo bean flours. While these also can be refined and processed, their quality and glycemic indices vary so it is important to read ingredients and nutritional index charts to learn more and know each food's value instead of assuming or eating blindly.

*Shop the **perimeter of the store** most of the time.* This is where we find most of the fresh quality fruits, vegetables, meats and refrigerated items. Usually the most nutrient-dense foods are found here. The inner aisles of a grocery store often contain the more processed prepackaged foods.

*Eat fewer **high glycemic** foods.* Refined, processed and simple carbohydrates are among the highest GI foods, e.g. bleached sugars and white flour products, overly refined and processed breads, pasta and baked goods.

*Eat more fruit and **whole fruit** with skin on, when possible, for extra fiber.* Pay attention to quality and quantity and limit fruit juices which have a higher sugar content and less fiber. Try eating fruit instead of sweets and/or desserts. Good examples include unsweetened applesauce and sliced fruits or a whole medium apple (approximately 10 grams sugar, 3 grams fiber with a GI of 38). Other good choices are raspberries, blackberries and strawberries (approximately 5-7 grams sugar, 3 grams fiber and GI of 40).

When attending a gathering or a pot luck, try bringing a fruit salad made of mostly berries, perhaps with a topping of vanilla Greek yogurt, instead of a sweet baked dessert. When eating fruits, make the berries and organic fruits with skin on your "go to" picks. These are more nutrient-dense and have less sugar and more fiber than melons or tropical fruits.

Remember that fruits vary in glycemic index, choose wisely and eat fewer high glycemic fruits by themselves. Some of the higher GI fruits include: pineapple with 16 grams of sugar per cup, grapes with 15 sugar grams per cup and 14 grams of sugar in one medium-sized banana. All of these range in the mid 50s for glycemic index.

Do not "throw the baby out with the bath water." Even though a fruit or vegetable may be of a higher glycemic value, do not negate its value. There are many fruits that have a medium to high glycemic index but also great nutritional and anti-inflammatory value. Pineapples and cherries are great examples.

A good habit is to combine these with lower GI foods like nuts or whole grain crackers and cheese.

*Minimize **sugary drinks**.* This includes pure unadulterated fruit juice beverages. Even though they may be natural, they generally have a high sugar content and are rated high GI. Avoid the obvious: fruit juices or prepackaged fruit that have added sugar (e.g. canned mandarin oranges, pears, apple sauce and pineapple). Buy organic when possible and without added sugar. Fruit juice sweetened is better, but beware of the actual sugar quantity in grams. It maddens me to see unnecessary sugar added to naturally sweet fruits!

*Consume **less sugar** in general.* Stop or at the very least, decrease consumption of soda and beverages with added sugar and or artificial sweeteners. Instead, try "*soda juice*" or a "*mocktail*" for a special drink. Simply take plain seltzer water, add a splash of pure fruit juice, frozen or fresh fruit or squeezed citrus and serve in a special glass to add to the fun factor.

*Avoid **higher GI sweeteners** and abstain from **artificial sweeteners**.* Learn about the variations in sugars and their place on the GI spectrum: stevia (0), agave syrup (15), brown rice syrup (25), honey (50), maple syrup (54) and blackstrap molasses (55). These are preferable to processed "fake" pancake syrup, white sugar and high fructose corn syrup, all of which fall in the high GI range.

Artificial sweeteners may have lower GI indices, but they are not always the best choices for our health or weight management. They can alter the sweetness taste buds, causing the desire and need for a more intense "hit" to satisfy the sweet tooth. They also create the false need for insulin because the body believes it took in sugar or glucose even though it did not. This leads to an increase in the craving for carbohydrates which, with excess use, can lead to any number of inflammatory illnesses.

Balance higher GI foods and simple carbohydrates by pairing them with lower GI foods. This might mean eating peanut butter and toast with a banana, cottage cheese with pineapple, or lean proteins on salad greens.

*Use **seeds** to add more fiber, quality protein and fat to your menus.* This can be achieved by adding fresh, whole or ground flax or chia seeds to salads, smoothies, cooked oatmeal, granola and even cookie recipes. Both seeds contain quality fat (omega-3s), protein and fiber. Chia is hardier, easier to keep fresh and a bit easier to digest. It can be stored at room temperature and does not need to be ground right before use or at all to maintain its nutrient value. Flax retains its value best if refrigerated and freshly ground just prior to each use. It also may be more difficult to digest than chia because of its lignin (a tough fiber).

Here is a comparison of what one tablespoon of each contains:

Flax seeds		Chia seeds
1 gram	**protein**	2 grams
2 grams	**fiber**	4 grams
2 grams	**omega-3 fatty acid**	1.75 grams

*Eat more **vegetables**.* Add an extra vegetable to a meal (greens, broccoli, asparagus or kale) instead of a starch (white rice, potatoes, chips or fries). Add a small side salad to a meal. Dare to be different or non-traditional. For example, it is perfectly fine to add a little sweet bibbed lettuce demi salad to the all-American egg breakfast.

Another way to up your vegetable content is to add a bit of zip to your simple lettuce-cucumber-tomato salad with shaved carrots or beets, finely chopped kale or red radishes. Enhance the less than nutritious iceberg or common romaine lettuce by mixing in some arugula, bok choy, red or green leaf lettuce. Even last night's leftover vegetables can be chopped into today's lunch or dinner salad.

*Ramp up the vegetable quality of your meals by adding more **nutrient dense** foods.* These are choices that contain the highest vitamin and mineral quotients per calorie. Nutrient density is a long standing term to measure the quality of certain foods. Depending on who is ranking the foods, a certain set of nutrients are being measured. There are a number of varied listings that can be accessed easily online.

One of the more familiar is from Dr. Joel Furhman MD, the originator of the *Nutritarian Diet*. He created the ANDI (Aggregate Nutrient Density Index) scale. This is a ranking of foods, primarily vegetables, on a scale from 1-1,000. The higher the number, the more nutrient dense the food is rated, based on 34 nutritional parameters. Fuhrman's goal is to help people achieve a high level of nutritional intake while ingesting fewer unnecessary calories. Examples of these ratings include some of our favorite cruciferous vegetables like kale (1,000), spinach (707), Brussels sprouts (490) and broccoli (340).

This is a very interesting and helpful concept to explore. I would highly recommend doing some online research if this data makes you curious or interested. It can be fun and inspiring to delve into the many lists of nutrient dense foods. Sometimes posting a list of these on the refrigerator can be helpful and inspiring.

Although accessing this type of information may be helpful and intriguing, there are many ways to improve the quality of vegetable and fruit intake without doing extra time-consuming research or depending on reference charts. Keep it simple! Make it easy to eat and live wellness as the next suggestions may prove.

*Eat a **variety** of fruits and vegetables.* Eating a broad spectrum assures the complete range of required nutrients. The various colors can be very helpful to achieve this. Notice the spectrum of what is consumed over the course of a day. Is there variety among food choices?

*Eat more **cruciferous** vegetables.* These are some of the most nutrient dense—kale, broccoli, Brussels sprouts, cauliflower, cabbage and dandelion, beet and Swiss chard greens.

*Eat fruits and vegetables that **grow in a variety** of ways.* For example, apples grow above ground, turnips grow below ground, grapes grow on vines, peas grow in pods, pears grow on trees and beans grow in bushes or on trellises and poles. These variations can carry different energies that are transferred to us.

*Notice how different foods bring about certain **feelings**.* Mood and energy and wellness can be directly affected by the foods we eat. Are they appealing? Do cravings increase after eating certain foods? What about cooking methods? Are steamed, broiled, boiled, roasted or raw most interesting? Try a variety of techniques and see how they feel. Different seasons and moods may bring about different appeal and wellness factors. Listen to the wise body and mind.

Ayurvedic and macrobiotic practices share the theory that foods have and promote certain energies. For example, upward growing fruits and vegetables (pineapple, lettuce, pole beans) bring more energy and lightness while downward growing and vine-grown foods (squash, onions, carrots) are more grounding and may even slow us down.

Different foods can have different values depending on their energies, and depending on our wellness, mood and the season, they may have different effects. *"Food is medicine."* This is a whole practice in and of itself and is quite fascinating. I encourage my clients to explore this concept if they find it appealing.

While the breadth and depth necessary for full understanding of this philosophy is beyond the scope of this book, I hope to spark some interest in readers and to introduce this concept because its value is remarkable. I often integrate this way of thinking into my personal and professional wellness practice. We all may notice that it is naturally occurring in our daily and seasonal habits more than we realize.

*Try eating food from **different climates**.* Notice what produce and dishes are appealing during certain seasons. Oftentimes hot tea drinks, soups and vegetables such as squash and root vegetables (carrots, parsnips, potatoes) are more appealing in the winter, especially when residing in cooler climates. In summer, the cooler drinks and foods (iced teas, salads, fresh fruits) are more appealing and agreeable to our system.

Local, in-season produce is often more easily digested and appealing. In this time of easy travel, people frequently live and travel far from their natural climates, eating foods foreign to their familiar habitats and cultures. Try to notice whether certain foods from different climates agree with the body-mind or leave you wanting more.

*Focus on **fresh and local** when possible.* The closer the vegetables and fruit are grown, the less time it takes them to reach our homes, giving the product less time to lose its nutritional value in transport. Depending on the product, the longer a food is exposed to air and bumped around, the more nutrients are lost.

Even organic products may not be as valuable as local, especially when they are imported from another country. It takes some of these foods weeks to arrive and various countries' organic standards do not equally compare to those of the U.S. Organic may have a varied quality across the globe. Even frozen vegetables can be of higher nutritional value than far travelled organic foods or products sitting in a store bin for an extended period of time.

Canned fruits and vegetables can be high in quality, but typically not the highest in nutritional value. Some food containers are made with harmful chemicals, including BPA (bisphenol A), which is used to line some cans and to make many types of plastic-ware. BPA can be a health hazard in high quantities, so it is best to avoid it as much as possible. If a can or plastic container does not say BPA-free, then it probably contains the product. Canned products often contain preservatives in the form of salt or sodium to help maintain freshness. Sugar can be another sneaky additive to be aware of in packaging.

Oftentimes, but not always, fresher foods are more natural in color and tend to be firmer to the touch. But do not be fooled by brilliant colors—sometimes foods raised with extra pesticides, insecticides and expedient growth elements can have been thusly altered from their natural form in order to make them more appealing and salable. For example, the most beautiful perfect tomato is not always the most healthy and nutrient dense or tasteful.

*Try different **cooking methods**.* These options also change in appeal with the seasons and the climate; we tend to eat more raw fresh foods in the summer and longer slow-cooked stews and soups in the winter. How a food is cooked can alter the energy or effect it has on our mind and body.

*When **eating out**, make a game of seeing how healthy and balanced a meal can be.* Order a simple salad or vegetable soup and eat this before a meal instead of bread, or order an extra side vegetable or a sweet potato to replace the ubiquitous white potato or French fries. Try an herbal or unsweetened black tea instead of a cocktail, soda, juice or sugary dessert. If it is a special occasion, however, do not be afraid to share a dessert and have a small taste (rather than the whole thing).

*Pay attention to **food ingredients**.* When eating a packaged food, look at what's in it, not just calories. Ingredients are listed in order of quantity in descending order. Notice what is listed first as this is the primary content. Is it sugar? Is it sugar by a different name, such as fructose, sucrose, corn syrup, etc.? Companies try to disguise sugar. Is it fruit juice sweetened or artificially sweetened with chemical sweeteners? If white or bleached enriched flour is one of the top ingredients, remember that white flour equals white sugar in the body and these tend to have a higher glycemic index.

Read **labels/nutrition facts**. Finding the truth about what we are eating with regard to quantity and quality can feel like trying to solve a riddle. And to complicate the job even more, food companies *try* to fool us into thinking something is healthy or natural by playing with words and numbers. "Natural" and "whole" do not always mean what they say. It pays to dig deeper into ingredient information.

Notice the specific nutrition facts on a label to determine the actual measures of certain elements:

- *Sugar.* Notice how many *total* grams of sugar the product contains. Even products without added sugar, e.g. natural fruit juices, can still have a high sugar content that affects blood sugar.

- *Carbohydrates:* This is also measured in grams, similar to sugar. While it is good to notice how many carbohydrates are in a food, these do not stand alone in determining overall GI or effects on blood sugar. Sometimes *net carbohydrates* are listed. This is the total carbohydrates minus the fiber, and is the more true carbohydrate value. Do the math to note the difference if it is not listed.

- *Fiber:* Notice how many grams of fiber are in the product. This number can cover a wide range. A greater number helps make for a lower GI. It is not essential to have fiber in everything we eat, but it is good to look for it in certain foods that should be high in fiber, such as crackers and bread. It is important to have daily fiber but everyone has different tolerances. More is not always better. Notice the response as more fiber is added to the daily diet. Does it cause bloating, gas or loose bowels? Introduce fiber gradually and modify the amount as needed for best tolerance. More natural or whole foods usually have more fiber and help balance blood sugar.

- *Protein.* More protein makes for a lower GI, but more is not always better. This is often best determined by lifestyle and body type. There is currently a great deal of hype around protein, but pay attention to how much is actually needed for different body types. Too much protein can stress the kidneys.

- *Serving size.* Do not be fooled! Sometimes this number is used to disguise excess sugar. Often we have to divide or multiply the amount listed in order to arrive at realistic measurements. Be sure to "do the math." Just because there are 10 crackers in a serving size, we do not have to eat all 10 crackers. Dividing by two can make a world of difference over time in health benefits. Similarly, who really eats a half-cup of cereal when the average breakfast bowl holds two cups?

When it comes to non-packaged, fresh foods such as fruits and vegetables, it is best to research online or in books some of the more commonly consumed food products. Notice the quantity and quality of important contents mentioned above, e.g. fiber, protein, sugar and fat.

Artificial sweeteners *are not natural and are typically chemicals that can be harmful to the body.* Although this may seem obvious, causing cancer is at the top of the ill-effects list for these products. Stevia and xylitol are currently two of the more natural sugar alternatives. They are both derived from plants, but they are still not ideal. There are many variations and alterations that make sugar replacements less natural, including how much they are processed. It is important to weigh the risks of sugar versus artificial sweeteners. If consuming alternative sweeteners, it is best to use them minimally and it is well worth trying to eliminate these entirely.

Green leaf stevia is the most natural sweetener, at 30 percent sweeter than table sugar. Next up is refined white stevia which is a whopping 200 percent sweeter than sugar. The least natural or most altered unnatural form of stevia goes by the brand name Truvia, and contains only 1 percent or less of the pure real stevia plant. The further we move from natural sweeteners, the more intense and exaggerated the sweet flavor becomes.

Most sweeteners are much sweeter to the taste than regular sugar, creating that craving for more we discussed above. Even bleached white sugar is sweeter than unaltered cane sugar (more brownish and natural in color). Sadly, the more sugar we take in, the less appealing and satisfying the natural sweetness of fruits and vegetables becomes.

Another natural alternative sweetener is xylitol. This substance can be more difficult to digest, causing a variety of possible digestive issues.

This can be bothersome even as an ingredient in *natural* chewing gum. It is best known for its dental benefits in preventing tooth decay. So, it is probably better used for oral hygiene as in a mouth rinse or in toothpaste rather than in food that is actually ingested.

Artificial sweeteners try to fake the body by adding a guiltless sweetness. Well worth repeating is the fact that, physiologically, they do just the opposite. The problem here is that the body thinks, when ingesting these sweeteners, that it has consumed glucose (when it hasn't) and releases insulin to process it. This causes cravings for more glucose, sugar and carbohydrates so it has something to actually process. A vicious cycle that fools no one.

*Eat at **regular intervals**.* If we go too long between meals, our blood sugar will drop. Then, depending on what we eat next, we are more likely to experience a greater spike, promoting the extreme rise and fall in glucose and insulin that feed inflammation. On average, it is best to eat every three to five hours. If we wait too long between meals, allowing excess hunger to creep in, we will be more apt to make poor food choices hastily or because we are "hangry."

On the other hand, eating too frequently, even in small amounts, is not good either. The body needs rest time from being in "digest" mode. It can be healthy to eat less food less often. My husband actually taught me that it's OK to leave food on my plate, even if it is just one last bite. It used to bother me to see food left on his plate, but over time I learned the value of this habit. The clean plate club is not one of the better groups to join.

*Feed your **sweet tooth**.* I know it sounds contradictory, but we all have some degree of need for sweets, and there are ways to add "sweetness" without turning exclusively to sugary foods. Yes, sugar-laden foods raise our "good feeling" endorphins, but so do less damaging sweet pleasures such as sweet potatoes, winter squashes, carrots and Vidalia onions. Fruits or herbal teas can also replace the indulges of candy and desserts.

It is even OK—healthy even—to enjoy a little dark chocolate, but be sure to pay attention to the ingredients. Make sure the chocolate is of high quality. This means it is organic, consists of no less than 60 percent cacao, contains little to no sugar (10 grams or less), and is made with cocoa butter rather than other oils (vegetable, palm, coconut). Cocoa butter is actually from the cacao bean and is not a dairy product.

Other sweet pleasures may have nothing to do with food. These include spending time in nature, sitting outside in the sunshine, going for a walk, taking a hike or going for a swim. Nature alone can be invigorating and raise endorphins. This makes most of us happy naturally.

Other suggestions:

- *Have fresh flowers* at home or in the workplace. We can buy flowers for ourselves. We do not have to wait for someone else to treat us.

- *Spend time with sweet people* who are fun or pleasing to be with. Make time to be with people who are admiring and loving. Others may think we are sweet, and that counts too if we enjoy their company.

- *Listen to sweet music*, something that lifts the spirits and brings pleasure, whether it be relaxing or reviving.

- *Enjoy art* that pleases the senses, either observing it or participating in its creation. Visit an art museum or gallery or attend a musical or athletic event. Play an instrument, sing or create art even if it is not highly skilled or accomplished. It can simply be for our own pleasure!

- *Move the body.* Dance, exercise. The fact that endorphins are released with activity has been proven over and over again. This is another form of sweetness. Sweating can be very good for us.

*Eat **mindfully*** and stimulate all the senses with food presentation. Here are some sweet tooth food and drink tricks:

- Eat slowly, "savor the flavor"

- Notice other senses such as texture and smell

- Use fancy or fun serving dishes, plates, bowls, tablecloths, napkins and festive glassware

- Jazz up the presentation by arranging food in a special way on the plate

- Eat by candlelight, outdoors or in a different location that feels special

- Garnish dishes with fresh herbs and fruit

- Thrill the taste buds with spices and natural flavors such as cinnamon on or in coffee with frothed milk or a dairy alternative

- Experiment with unfamiliar natural spices

- Drink homemade herbal or fruit-added and infused water

- Splash a bit of lemon juice in drinking water or plain seltzer

- Sweeten homemade lemonade and lower its GI by using a natural sweetener such as maple syrup

- Dilute juices and other sweet beverages with water or seltzer

Last but not least, we need to be kind and sweet ourselves for if we are, these qualities will come back to us.

*Learn to **socialize without overindulging** in continuous unhealthy pleasures.* Learn to say no thank you and know how to alter treats for social occasions. This means attending social gatherings without feeling pressured to eat and drink everything that is provided. Sometimes we feel guilty if we do not try the host's chocolate cake or drink wine all night with them. We need to take care of ourselves in this situation. We are the ones who have to live with the headache, broken sleep, guilt or sinus headache that we might wake up with.

*It's what we do **most** of the time, not just some of the time.* It is perfectly OK to have a little cake at a birthday party, but maybe not on everyone's birthday or not a giant piece. Some work places have birthday cake and celebrations often. Choose when to eat the treats and do not feel obliged to participate every time a cake or donuts or homemade treat shows up.

It is OK and important to socialize and gather with friends and family, but maybe not so good to overindulge with food and beverages every time people gather. Try one of the "mocktails" we mentioned earlier in these situations when choosing not to imbibe. Simply mix seltzer water with fresh lemon, lime or orange juice or maybe a splash of unsweetened cranberry or tart cherry juice; then add frozen fruit and pour the mixture into a fancy glass or stemware similar to the barware the other guests are using. Sometimes it feels better not to draw attention or to stand out.

Relationships and human interaction have been proven to be advantageous to health and wellness. It is okay to decline social gatherings, but not if it comes to avoiding *all* events. We need to find our own comfort zone and social groups that meet our needs for wellness. Notice what groups we *hang* with most and assess if it is enhancing or challenging our wellness.

*Change the **mindset**.* We tell ourselves "we deserve it," we had a long week or a hard day; life sucks, and we need a treat. Heeding these prompts *on occasion* is not harmful, but making them into life-long habits can be. Do we deserve the poor sleep, headaches, lack of energy, obsession or distraction, extra weight, anxiety or whatever else we experience with a poor diet? We could even take it to the next level of the undeserved and undesirable illnesses like glucose intolerance, pre-diabetes, high cholesterol, hypertension and a myriad of other illnesses and diseases. Let's rethink what we "deserve." Good sleep, steady consistent moods and energy, good health and a healthy weight— these are what we truly deserve.

Know the body *and its needs.* Figure out if we fall into one or more of these categories:

- ***Addict.*** If you are truly addicted to food or alcohol or some other substance, it is not realistic or even possible to eat just one cookie or dessert, drink the occasional cup of wine, smoke a cigarette and stop, enjoy one small coffee, or numb ourselves with whatever treat that calls us, without winding up bingeing. It is important to be honest when considering my suggested 90:10 guideline. Maybe abstinence from certain substances is best. It is important to know and honor our personal makeup of specific needs and tendencies. We are responsible for our self-care. Although not ill-intentioned, people do not always have our best interests in mind when they continually invite us for drinks or ice cream, and it is up to us to find other, healthier ways to connect with friends—take a walk, see a movie, have a cup of tea or a cool natural beverage. If you suspect that you are a food addict, there are some great support groups to explore, including Overeaters Anonymous (OA) and Food Addicts Anonymous (FAA). There also are professionals and health care practitioners who specialize in treating eating disorders. Try to find an appropriate way to break a cycle or bad habit and get a fresh start. Ask for help and get support.

- **Medical Patient.** Is there a medical issue brewing? Persistent symptoms of some sort that are not subsiding? Medical attention may be necessary to help manage the condition. If so, do not hesitate to contact your primary care physician, and do not leave any hints of illness unaddressed. Maybe there is a clear diagnosis, e.g. diabetes or heart disease. Be sure to work with specialized medical professionals to best understand your illness and how to manage it.

- **Athlete.** Athletes have a greater tolerance for eating higher GI foods. Extremely active people often need carbohydrates for quick energy and recovery, but if we fall into this category, it is important to pay attention if activity levels change and not train the taste buds for bad habits. Many highly muscular athletes end up deconditioned and overweight in their later years due to living the same high-calorie and often low-quality diet after their level of athleticism has changed.

- **Youth.** Younger people can typically handle higher GI foods. They are better able to process them because youngsters are typically more active, but they may be developing life-long habits and acquiring tastes that will eventually catch up with them. By eating sugary processed foods, kids can acquire a habitual taste and desire for them. It is important to feed children well and help them develop a palate for high-quality, nutrient-dense foods along with an active lifestyle.

- **Elderly.** Aging bodies tend to have more inflammation due to years of wear and tear and from processing foods and toxins. Naturally, our bodies become tired and actually wear out over time. Remember the catchy term *"inflammaging."* This occurs naturally with age so it is even more critical to eat a balanced glycemic index diet to prevent excess inflammation and aging processes in our bodies.

- ***Average.*** People of average weight, age and wellness who are trying to manage their health and prevent illness and disease do best by practicing a 90:10 lifestyle. Adopting and maintaining healthy habits is essential to the maintenance of wellness.

Understanding and applying what we know about glycemic index does not guarantee we will be well. GI is more like an important puzzle piece in the bigger picture of how to gain and maintain good health. A helpful tool for managing inflammation and promoting health as well as a useful guideline for choosing more quality foods. For example, here is a sample diet plan for one day based on balancing GI rankings.

- 7 am Breakfast: oatmeal with a handful of nuts or seeds and blueberries, or whole wheat toast with fresh tomatoes and avocado chunks drizzled with olive oil, squeezed lime and a pinch of sea salt

- 9:30 am Snack: plain Greek yogurt with granola

- 12 noon Lunch: salad with mixed vegetables and chicken

- 3 pm Snack: celery with peanut butter, goat cheese or hummus, or a cup of vegetable soup

- 6 pm Dinner: salmon, sweet potato and broccoli

- 8 pm snack: sliced pear and a small handful of nuts

Remember that there are quality nutrient-dense foods in the high glycemic category (like fruits), while there also are not so healthy choices in the low glycemic group (like excess fatty red meat). Compare the values. Do the positives outweigh the negatives? If not, then try to make a better choice, or simply minimize the frequency of consuming the lower quality foods and drinks.

Also, know that we could have a nicely balanced GI diet or meal but still be missing out on some key nutrients, e.g. eating meat and grains but no vegetables.

If this discussion of glycemic Index has piqued interest, go ahead and read and research more. The next level of information concerns something called *glycemic load*, which is how the amount and type of certain carbohydrates affect the timing of their release into the bloodstream. If formulas, details, data, equations and learning about glycemic load are interesting, maybe the next step is to advance your nutritional education.

There is always another level of learning. Just when we learn a little, we realize there is so much more to digest (pun intended). As we learn about improving our diet by adding more fruits and vegetables and eliminating unhealthy items, we can also move to the next level of learning. We may start to focus on questions such as which fruits and vegetables are the best? How do we prepare, cook and serve foods for the maximum bang for our nutritional buck? Which combinations work to optimize our overall physical health? Ideally, I would like to see all of us inspired to continue gaining nutritional knowledge and improve our diets for optimal health.

It is also important to keep things simple and doable. A minor little wholesome modification is always better than none at all. Healthy *sustainable* shifts work better in the long run. Starting small and being good to ourselves is more important than striving for perfection.

Remember, "It is what we do most of the time, not just some of the time." Think 90:10. Ninety percent of the time, if we eat well, we can let ourselves have a treat on occasion 10 percent of the time. Feeling deprived and bummed out has its own negative effects on our health.

Chapter 4: Digestion and Healthy Habits

As we continue to choose the proper foods for wellness, we also need to learn how to best digest them. Next, we will move on to another piece of the puzzle and learn how digestion and inflammation can interface and impact our health.

Digestion in the human body encompasses "start to finish," "entrance to exit" or "stem to stern." The process starts as soon as food or drink enters the mouth and ends with elimination, as the waste product exits in the form of urine or fecal matter.

A lot happens from beginning to end, and that makes plenty of room for error. With all the different processes occurring along the digestive path, inflammation and malfunctions can happen at numerous points. Remember the inflammatory markers and symptoms we talked about earlier? Digestive dysfunctions can have some of the same negative effects leading to illness and disease.

Let's review the steps in the process of digestion so we can make sense of some of the possible areas for breakdown.

The first steps begin when we simply start to think about food. Gastric juices start releasing within the digestive tract. Digestion becomes more active when we actually place food within the **mouth.** Food starts to break down with the chewing process and the release of digestive juices in the saliva or salivary juices. Hydrochloric acid and salivary amylase help start the breakdown of glucose or starch particles. Chewing is essential in order for nutrients to be released, become more digestible, and be accessible for the body to utilize for energy and system operations.

As food passes through the **esophagus** into the **stomach**, it churns with more digestive and acidic enzymes to continue breaking down. With a low pH of 1.5 - 2, this acidic environment aids in this process and allows for easier absorption. These early phases of digestion are important for the elimination of unwanted bacteria and microorganisms to help prevent illness and toxins from entering the rest of the body. Also in the stomach, protease is released to begin the process of breaking down protein.

When food particles are sufficiently processed by the stomach, they are passed into the **small intestine**. In the first part of the small intestine, the duodenum, most of the chemical digestion occurs. The **pancreas** secretes insulin and other digestive enzymes to help breakdown proteins (protease), carbohydrates (amylase) and fats (lipase).

The **liver** releases bile into the duodenum and

stores excess in the **gall bladder**. The liver and the gall bladder both connect to the small intestine through bile ducts. Bile has a very important role in digestion. It works to help digest fats with the enzyme lipase, kills unwanted bacteria and neutralizes the pH with bicarbonate ions before entering the latter parts of the small intestine. A more alkaline environment is created here at a pH level ranging between 7 and 8.

The liver also acts as a filter to the nutrients being absorbed through the small intestine. These nutrients arrive at the liver through the portal vein. The liver has a huge job in digestion and health. I like to think of it as the chemical engineering plant, as it helps detoxify chemicals, additives, preservatives, drugs, etc., either holding, releasing or processing as needed. The liver releases its own chemicals to process what it can. Normally, the liver returns waste products to the small intestine through bile or directly into the blood and lymphatic systems, leading to elimination through sweat or to the kidneys for urination. If waste is excessive, the liver may become overtaxed, causing dysfunction and sluggish performance.

The liver prioritizes jobs and oftentimes excess products waiting to be managed get recirculated until the liver can attend to them. Meanwhile, this causes the rest of the body to become exposed to toxins and excess fat and sugar. This is another good reason to minimize toxic elements from our diets.

Toxic load is a term often mentioned in natural diet and lifestyle. It refers to toxins and chemicals we may be exposed to through what we ingest or come in contact with in our environment. Decreasing our toxic load by eating and living clean can help decrease the taxing effects on our liver and other detox organs to improve health and help prevent illness and disease.

Extra byproducts of fat, glucose and toxins can remain in the liver, causing dysfunction or a buildup in other areas of the body. Many toxins are stored in fat throughout the body. Yet another reason to maintain a healthy weight to minimize excess fat stores in conjunction with eating clean and balancing glycemic index.

Some of the toxins released in the body are what we call "free radicals." These are incomplete atoms that can cause cell damage and in excess, lead to inflammation, disease and illness.

As the food moves through the rest of the small intestine (jejunum and ilium), most of the nutrients are absorbed into the bloodstream through the villi (small folds in the intestinal walls). The total length of the small intestine may be as much as 22 feet.

The **large intestine,** also known as the **colon**, removes extra water from what's left of the undigested food before it is excreted as waste in the form of stool or feces. Fiber is a friend for promoting a healthy colon. Fiber helps absorb toxins, bad bacteria and extra water. This helps keep the colon healthy by slowing digestion, lowering sugar levels, and ensuring the formation of normal bowel movements while preventing constipation and diarrhea.

The colon has three sections. The **ascending** colon runs from the front of the right hip up under the corner of the ribs. The **transverse** colon runs across the mid-torso from right to left. And the **descending** colon travels from under the front left corner of the ribs down to the front left hip area. The large intestine totals approximately 6 feet before it reaches the **rectum**. The average diameter of the colon is 3 inches.

The large intestine houses good and bad bacteria. Good bacteria in the gut fights infection, eats bad gut bacteria, supports the immune system and helps balance inflammation. Bacteria wants to ferment and grow and multiply, so these organisms will capitalize on what we feed them. Bad bacteria thrive on red meat, sugar, simple carbs and excess glucose. Good bacteria likes prebiotics, probiotics and fermented foods.

Bowel and Bladder Health

A person's elimination can tell us a lot about their level of wellness. The ideal, normal or optimal frequency for bowel movement is 1-2 times per day, with stools that are softly formed like toothpaste, sausage shaped and produced with a minimum of effort. Frequency norms may vary from person to person ranging up to once every two days. If stool floats, it may mean that fat is not being properly digested. If it sinks, fat is typically being digested adequately.

As for bladder health, a few basics can be very helpful in understanding and self-assessing. Normal bladder function is urinating approximately every 2-4 hours. Color and odor can be indicators or helpful hints of proper hydration. Normal is similar in color to light yellow lemonade and without significant odor. If the urine is darker or more odorous, this can be a sign of dehydration or even the start of an infection. Dehydration can cause increased urine concentration and bladder irritation. This may also lead to increased urgency and frequency, inflammation, and even infection and incontinence. Poor digestion or an imbalanced diet and lifestyle can also influence these detoxification systems.

Anywhere along this long chain of digestion, dysfunction can occur leading to inflammation, illness and disease.

Some basic **signs and symptoms** of imbalance, inflammation or poor digestive health include:

- Canker sores
- Bad breath
- Heartburn and indigestion
- Belching and burping
- Bloating and fluid retention
- Nausea and vomiting
- Frequent urination, incontinence and changes in bladder health
- Gas, flatulence, diarrhea and constipation

Other less obvious signs of inflammation or trouble with digestion can include:

- Fatigue, sluggishness or low energy
- Short temperedness or excessive anger (Practitioners of traditional Chinese medicine say that the "liver is off" when excess anger or out of character anger occurs.)
- Cellulite, weight gain or weight loss
- Trouble gaining or losing weight
- Rash or skin irritations or breakouts (e.g. acne or liver spots; skin is a backup elimination organ to the bowel and bladder)
- Congestion, excess phlegm or mucous
- Coughing or sneezing

- Swollen and/or red eyes and yellow eyes
- Headache
- Trouble concentrating, brain fog, depression or anxiety
- Blood sugar imbalances (hypo/hyperglycemic)
- PMS, menstrual dysfunction or fertility issues
- Sleep disturbances
- Hair loss
- Musculoskeletal pain

If any of the above symptoms are occurring, it may be helpful to review them with a health care practitioner. Reading on into the next chapter can be useful to improve digestion too. Try a few simple tricks to see if they help.

<u>Chapter 5: Supporting Good Digestion</u>

The easiest way to approach the important topic of digestion is to focus on suggestions in an orderly manner. To help simplify the process, I have organized the following recommendations in the order in which digestion occurs—from the beginning to the end or top to bottom.

While reading through this information, think about choosing only one or two action items to practice for a week or two. Then, reassess the effects experienced. Is there a change in any unwanted symptoms? How is your energy level? Mental clarity? Bowels, bladder function, weight, etc.? Next, decide whether or not to continue with the same action item or whether a tweak may be necessary for another week or two trial. Maybe decide on another item or two. Keep it simple and constant for success!

Getting Started

My favorite place to begin improving digestive health is with awareness of the need to balance the **Autonomic Nervous System** (ANS). This is the part of the nervous system that houses the Parasympathetic Nervous System (PNS) and the Sympathetic Nervous System (SNS). Of the two, it is the Parasympathetic Nervous System that is most relevant to good digestion. It is known for "rest and digest" and "rest and recover." Our focus will be on the digest mode. If this is in tune and active, then we are able to digest our food more easily and our organs are able to do their job and function optimally.

The Sympathetic Nervous System is best known as the area where "fight or flight" occurs. This is the mode that is important and most active when we are in danger. Although we may not always be in a true state of emergency, we spend a lot of our time in this condition. In our busy lives, we carry on all revved up and this sets us up for trouble.

This ongoing stress can play an active part in ruining our sleep as well as our digestion, leaving us exhausted by a higher level of resting tension. This can then result in slower healing and increased pain if we are injured. The SNS causes an increased release of cortisol and adrenaline. These are hormones that, in excess, have been proven to play a part in increasing inflammation. As we noted in earlier chapters, this correlation is extremely relevant to increased illness and disease.

It is essential to support both the PNS and the SNS for an ideal digestive climate. Listed below are a few ways to do that. Try to notice which techniques resonate and then implement those suggestions each day as much as possible.

- Sit down when eating, and focus directly on the meal or snack.

- Avoid eating "on the run," while standing in the kitchen, or when driving.

- Take a few relaxing breaths to transition into digestion mode as chewing begins.

- Practice relaxation techniques such as meditation or mindfulness regularly, before, during and after mealtimes as well as at various times throughout the day.

- Try a smart phone app to help with meditation and relaxation.

Keep Breathing

Diaphragmatic breathing is an especially simple yet profound technique that has a direct effect on the nervous system as a whole. The diaphragm and the ANS are both regulated by the vagus nerve, which manages the release of acetylcholine. This, in turn, stimulates the release of cortisol. Although essential in many ways, these are both known as stress hormones. In excess they can cause an imbalance in the ANS by facilitating an increase in the SNS.

I have created a 20-minute guided relaxation session titled "Pause & Breathe." It uses a series of contract-relax exercises followed by a sequence of focused breath work. This can be accessed through my website, business Facebook page or LinkedIn accounts. See (links in the resources section at the end of this book.)

Learning diaphragmatic or "barrel breathing" is simple and need not be complicated. It involves taking a full, relaxing breath, allowing the belly or lower torso to rise and expand, then exhaling while letting the belly relax and retract. Simply imagine the ribs and trunk like a barrel, fill the barrel with air, watch it expand, then slowly let it empty.

Adding a count to the inhale, pause and exhale can be helpful in monitoring the breath and maximizing the effects. The rate varies depending on the practitioner. I have used a variety and have found a count of four to be most simple. Breathe in for a count of four, pause for a count of four then out for a count of four, pause for a count of four and repeat for four cycles four times a day or whenever needed or reminded. Specifically breathing in through the nose and out through the nose or mouth also varies from practitioner to practitioner. I find each helpful at different times. Try a variety and see what feels right.

For optimal effects, many wellness practitioners recommend that this type of breathing exercise be done frequently, throughout the day. I like to remind people to practice this when they feel revved up or in conjunction with other routine activities like approaching a stop sign or going to the bathroom. Most important is to take a full relaxing breath before each meal.

A few other suggestions for approaching each meal with good digestion in mind:

- Focus and remain as calm as possible.

- Eat slowly and with attention to the miraculous process of eating and digesting.

- Avoid stressful conversations, whether personal or work-related.

- Limit brain stimulating activities like TV, computer work and gaming while eating.

Using these tools will foster healthy digestion by putting the body in a relaxed state of mind and maximizing the functioning of the PNS. These techniques may also help diminish the swallowing of air, which can cause belching or even nausea.

With drinks in mind:

Once we master the process of eating, we need to pay attention to drinking and the **fluids** we drink around mealtimes. How can they affect digestion? What types and timing of beverages can promote or impede digestive functioning?

A few suggestions:

- Start a meal with warm fluids like soup, warm water (with or without lemon), decaffeinated herbal or green tea. Warm fluids before a meal can prepare for optimal digestion and aid in relaxation of the system, both physically and mentally. The warmth can be calming and helps dilate and promote circulation in the digestive tract.

- Avoid cold liquids close to meals. Iced beverages are not friendly to digestion and absorption. Cold fluids around mealtimes can be constricting and cause a more rigid digestive tract, impairing digestion. When eating out, it is okay to ask for water without ice.

- Avoid excess fluids with a meal, to avoid diluting digestive juices. Too much liquid can alter the pH (degree of acidity) of the gastric fluids needed for digestion. On a scale of 0-14, acidic to basic, stomach acid has an acidic pH of approximately 1.9. Water is more basic at approximately 7 or greater, which is too alkaline or basic in pH and can impede the digestive process.

Food that passes through less digested decreases absorption of quality nutrients and causes stress to the latter parts of the digestive process, i.e., the large intestine. This can also cause discomfort, increased gas and bloating. Hydration is very important, but it is better to drink water or fluids between meals rather than during.

- Consider drinking just one or two tablespoons of apple cider vinegar or water with lemon juice in warm or room temperature water just before or after a meal. (This is one liquid that it is OK to sip during a meal.) Both of these fluids have pH levels similar to the body's digestive enzymes. Not only are they helpful with basic digestion, but they can also help bile function to kill bacteria and assist the cleansing of the gall bladder, preventing gallstones.

- Use lemon juice to aid digestion, detoxify and stimulate liver function, and stabilize free radicals in the bloodstream, but when slicing or juicing lemons, *always wash them first!* Better still, buy organic lemons when possible. I often wonder if restaurants wash those lemons that they drop into our drinks. Sometimes, I ask for lemons served on the side, so I can squeeze them myself and discard the rind.

- Drink plenty of filtered or purified water (again, between meals). This will reduce the need for filtering by the liver. A qualified water company or even an over-the-counter test kit can easily determine the quality of tap water. A water purifier or a simple container such as a Brita filtering pitcher can help remove unwanted impurities.

- Try to drink 6-8 glasses of water per day. Fruits and vegetables, soups and non-caffeinated herbal teas count toward this level of hydration.

- Facilitate good hydration habits, by keeping easily accessible cups in the bathroom. Starting the day with a cup of water is ideal. A good habit is to drink water upon rising in the morning or soon after brushing our teeth. We can think of morning water as a shower for the inside body, much like the shower we take for the outside body. Dr. Shawn Stevenson calls this the "inner bath."

This emphasis on hydrating properly early in the day is important because the body is often dehydrated first thing in the morning. Much of the water in our system is used during the night's rest and recovery state. Our first fluids have a great influence on all of our organs, muscles and tissues. If coffee is our first beverage, we can be doing our body a great disservice. If immediate AM coffee is essential, at least try drinking an 8-ounce glass of water first.

Because our bodies are made up of 60 percent water, and we depend on this to help maintain an efficient digestive system, a good rule of thumb is to take in half our body weight in ounces of fluid each day. For a 200-pound person, that would be 100 ounces or a little more than three quarts of water or clear fluids per day. For most of us, getting even four glasses of water per day would be great progress!

To conclude, dehydration can cause many symptoms in the body. These include hunger, fatigue, headaches, dizziness, poor mental clarity, constipation and bladder irritation.

We Are How We Eat

There are many suggestions for how to aid the digestive process by choosing the right foods and ingesting them correctly. It sounds obvious, but many of us need to think about something as basic as chewing. Here are a few tips and a few of my thoughts on how to continue to aid digestion and decrease or prevent inflammation.

- Avoid sending un-chewed or barely chewed food to the stomach. Focus on chewing until no solids remain, turning food to mush with the consistency of baby food. If it is helpful, think about why we feed babies pureed food—because babies have no teeth. But we do, so it is important to use them!

- Proper chewing can decrease the amount of gas and bloating we experience by helping with digestion and absorption early in the digestive process. Poorly digested food can lead to gas later in the colon where it reacts with bad gut bacteria. Food is meant to be chewed for optimal absorption.

- Smoothies are great but only on occasion, as they eliminate the need for chewing. This can cause fewer digestive juices to be released for processing. And they are often cold, which is also constricting. My most-loved winter version of a hot smoothie is soup. (Dairy-free autumn bisque is one of my favorites.)

- As mentioned earlier, cooler beverages and foods are better in the warmer seasons while warmer liquids are optimal during cooler months. There is great value in learning about "eating with the seasons." A great start to doing that is to listen to our bodies and notice how our desires for different foods and temperatures change with the seasons.

I once attended a class titled "Love your Liver." One of my long-time favorite teachers supporting *food is medicine* is Lisa Silverman who taught cooking classes and theories about macrobiotics. She often did seasonal classes to teach about the five-element theory, eating with the seasons and supporting the primary body systems and organs. This is amazing information, and I strongly suggest researching more of this Eastern philosophy for a greater understanding of how to support our bodies' natural tendencies. A book by Nelson M. Haas, *Staying Healthy with the Seasons,* is a great reference.

Other influences on this topic—and on my life!—are Warren Kramer and Meg Wolff. They too specialize in macrobiotics and have taught a number of classes where I learned to expand my palate and knowledge of vegan eating and seasonal awareness.

- Choose a plant-based diet. Fruits and vegetables support liver function and aid digestion on many levels.

- Eat a variety of colors to get a full spectrum of nutrients. The rich colors in vegetables and fruits are called **flavonoids**. Some great examples are dark green vegetables like broccoli, kale, Brussels sprouts, orange carrots and squash, red tomatoes, beets and blueberries.

- Go for fiber-rich foods. These tend to be low on the glycemic index scale. They help clean the digestive tract by attaching themselves to bad bacteria, fats and other toxins which are evacuated with bowel movements. Fiber is like an internal vacuum cleaner or the body's very own Pac Man.

- Eat foods high in antioxidants to help prevent and eliminate free radicals that can cause cell damage and lead to illness and disease. Antioxidants inhibit the oxidation or deterioration of nutrients in foods we eat. Some of the higher antioxidant foods and spices are kale, carrots, blueberries, dark chocolate (at least 70 percent cacao), cinnamon, parsley, ginger, garlic and green tea. The list is extensive and worth exploring.

In some of my research, Dr. Shawn Stevenson remarks on early medical studies by a variety of doctors, including the late Henry A. Mattill, that "animals eating whole foods lived longer and remained healthier." Vitamins C and E were some of the earliest antioxidant elements discovered. Please note, this is not a reason to simply take supplements. Eating real whole foods is more often beneficial, unless supplements are recommended by our medical practitioner.

- Add anti-inflammatory spices, such as turmeric or curry, to everyday meals. These often contain polyphenols which are micronutrients that have been shown to help prevent degenerative diseases. Try some Indian food, or add cinnamon to oatmeal, coffee or tea.

- Eat kale for so many reasons! Not only is this green a super anti-inflammatory food, it is great for detoxing the body due to its high sulfur content. And there are many ways to add it to our diets. Try putting it in scrambled eggs with sautéed onions and garlic. Or, soften it with a touch of sea salt and lemon and add it to a salad. Kale chips can easily be made by baking the leaves (trim off the stems) with a touch of sea salt. To make what is called "massaged" kale (easier to digest than raw kale), simply wash and chop the leaves, place them in a bowl, and squeeze on the juice of half a lemon. Add a dash of sea salt and massage with fingertips until the kale softens. Let sit for 5-10 minutes then squeeze and remove excess lemon juice.

- Incorporate seaweed. Like kale, seaweed "has it all," a low glycemic index score, high fiber, protein, and omega-3 fatty acids, plus, anti-viral, anti-oxidant and anti-inflammatory effects. Seaweed is also high in calcium and many other nutrients, and has been known to aid in liver and blood detoxification, especially from heavy metals. (We have all been exposed to more than we realize—lead, aluminum, and the mercury in tooth fillings, water and fish.)

The only thing to keep in mind about seaweed is that more is not always better since it is high in sodium and iodine. Be cautious in its use, especially with hyperthyroidism. To use, measure one square inch per cup of water when adding it to soup, beans or brown rice. Discard from the beans after they are cooked, to decrease gassiness by breaking down extra fiber.

A few types of seaweed are nori, wakame, kombu, arame and dulce. Nori comes in sheets and is used to roll sushi. I use kombu or wakame in soups, beans and brown rice. Dulce is very good on salads after soaking it in filtered water.

Good digestion requires that we focus on ingesting **phytochemicals** or **phytonutrients.** These are compounds found in plants that make them unique, for example, the smell of garlic, the sting of onions or the rich colors of fruits and vegetables. Their primary purpose is to protect and sustain the plants as they grow, but evidence is gaining that their health benefits for humans as antioxidants help prevent illness and promote wellness. These plant gems can be very helpful in aiding the prevention of early degenerative diseases of the eyes and heart, and even cancer.

Carotenoids are one of the better known groups of phytochemicals:

- Orange vegetables like carrots contain *beta carotene*, which the body converts to vitamin A to support healthy eyes, skin, hair, nerves, and heart and brain functioning.

- Green vegetables like spinach and Swiss chard contain *lutein*, which is also known for benefiting the eyes, the skin and the heart.

- Red tomatoes, pink grapefruits and watermelons contain *lycopene* which can be helpful to skin and cardiac health.

- Pineapple contains *bromeliad,* a natural anti-inflammatory.

- Tart cherries are high in vitamins A and C, and *melatonin* which regulates the body's sleep-wake cycles.

- Apples contain *pectin,* an insoluble fiber that binds to fats and cholesterol and heavy metals, assisting the liver in the detoxification process.

- Red apples and red onions contain *quercetin* which has been shown to decrease allergies, asthma and to improve heart health.

- Beets and beet greens are good for toning and rebuilding the liver for they contain *betaine*, a natural liver detoxifier and bile thinner. In turn, this aids the liver in digesting fats. Beets are excellent grated with a little lemon juice or boiled and sliced onto a salad.

- Garlic helps activate liver enzymes through *selenium* and *allicin.* It also contains *methionine,* an amino acid that helps eliminate toxins into the urine.

Another thing to pay attention to with regard to good digestion is the quality of fats. *Unsaturated* fats are best, like monounsaturated (avocado and olive), and polyunsaturated (salmon, walnuts, almonds, seeds). Although it is possible to take these in the form of supplements, I recommend ingesting these nutrients with real foods instead. Bioavailable nutrients are easier to digest and for the body to absorb and utilize for health purposes.

My favorite oils are olive, avocado and coconut. Different oils retain or lose their nutritional value at different temperatures. For example, coconut oil maintains the quality of its omega-3 value better than many other oils when used for cooking at higher temperatures. Olive oil is better at room temperature and is particularly good on salad. At higher temperatures, some oils actually create free radicals adding to our *toxic load.*

What Not to Eat

Now that we have discussed all the good foods we should be eating, let us take a look at those to be avoided or at least minimized.

- Avoid toxins, pesticides, chemicals, heavy metals and artificial ingredients and colors. These can build up in the body causing extra work for the liver as well as cell damage that can lead to illness and disease.

- Limit consumption of the larger, predatory fish at the top of the food chain, such as swordfish, shark and tuna. (Albacore is an exception, which is younger tuna and less toxic.) The smaller and typically younger fish at the bottom of the food chain, for example, salmon, crab, sardines or trout are cleaner fish. The larger, older fish have had years to absorb toxins, and they eat many smaller fish and plankton causing an additional accumulation of toxins and mercury.

- Try to steer clear of farm-raised fish unless the fish farm is well known for its clean practices. Is the living area large or are the fish sharing a smaller, more toxic space that is minimally oxygenated and filled with fish waste? Are the fish fed antibiotics and pesticides? Are they fed fish meal and products to expedite growth? Is coloring added to make the fish more appealing? Ask *where* and *how* questions about the fish we buy and eat.

As for wild-caught fish, ask where it was fished since not all bodies of water are equal in cleanliness. Typically, wild ocean fish are cleaner than lake, pond or stream caught fish. Larger, colder bodies of water tend to be cleaner than smaller and warmer waters, where the density of toxins and bacteria are more prevalent.

The Environmental Protections Agency (EPA) is a good source of information about the safety of edible fish. The EPA reports annually on test results from studies of bodies of water as well as fish.

Both the USDA and the non-profit Environmental Working Group (EWG) have proven in a number of studies that farm-raised fish contain higher toxins and a lower percentage of nutrients than wild caught.

- Stay away from GMOs (genetically modified organisms). These are food products that have been created in a laboratory, where their genetics are altered in order to make them easier to mass produce at a lower cost. Corn and soy are two of the most commonly genetically modified foods. Be sure that foods are labelled *non-GMO,* or even better, *organic.* Although there have been mixed reports on the effect of GMOs on the body, ask what is the source of the report. Are they associated with the (manufacturing) plants or the (vegetable garden) plants?

- Limit the use of *all* artificial ingredients (sweeteners, dyes, flavorings and preservatives such as MSG or monosodium glutamate), or any food that is overly processed. All of these toxins can be stored as free radicals in the body, leading to inflammation and illness. The best foods come from nature, not factories.

- Be aware of unhealthy fats. These include saturated fats, trans fats, hydrogenated fats and partially hydrogenated fats. These are the types most often found in margarine, fried foods, baked goods, processed and prepackaged foods, and animal products such as red meat and chicken skin.

  These products increase LDLs, also known as bad cholesterol. Excess bad fats dumped into the body and bloodstream can cause high cholesterol and be stored throughout the body, "clogging up the system."

  A few exceptions to the evil reputation of saturated fats are unrefined coconut oil, organic butter and ghee (clarified butter). Although these are saturated fats, they are more easily digested by the body and in their most pure form can aid in balancing glycemic index and minimizing sugar spikes.

Even cooking with some oils at very high temperatures can cause problems. These oils can oxidize under those conditions, become free radicals, and promote cancer.

- With regard to *alcohol*—a beverage that deserves a bit of extra attention—a good rule of thumb is to avoid it more often than not, since it is one of the most taxing products on the liver. Alcohol is one of the few products that is immediately absorbed through the stomach into the bloodstream. From there it is sent directly to the liver.

  The liver is a smart organ. It prioritizes what it processes, and knows that alcohol is a poisonous substance that needs to be taken care of first. Alcohol can interfere with digestion as it may take precedence over other elements to be processed. This may lead to additional toxins getting through the system or not properly being filtered by the liver.

Alcohol dehydrogenase (ADH) is one of the primary enzymes that metabolizes alcohol. It is secreted primarily in the stomach, but also in the liver, where most of the alcohol is processed. Alcohol has to be converted to acid aldehyde or acetaldehyde in order to be excreted. If we do not produce enough dehydrogenase to process the alcohol, then there will be an accumulation of this toxin that then acts like a poison.

This toxin can accumulate and be stored in fat, in the liver, or in other parts of the body, leading to weight gain, illness, inflammation and dysfunction in the digestive process. Alcohol can cause a basic hangover or severe illness. Excess undigested alcohol can lead to symptoms that may include headache, dizziness, lightheadedness, nausea, vomiting or even alcohol poisoning or death. Different people have different tolerances or abilities to process alcohol, and this should be respected.

Acetaldehyde is also a known carcinogen and, over time, in large amounts can lead to cancer. Most health care guidelines therefore recommend imbibing only one to two drinks per day and none with a personal risk for any form of cancer.

Even if we allow one or two drinks a day we can be interfering with the direct health of our liver and life expectancy. The benefits touted by some professionals do not outweigh the ill effects. In fact, new research shows that even as little as one drink per day increases the chance of getting breast cancer by 5-10 percent, depending on one's age.

The more we drink, the higher our risk for a variety of cancers. One of the earliest reports confirming alcohol consumption's correlation to cancer was published in 1987 by the World Health Organization (WHO). More recently the American Society of Clinical Oncology (ASCO) issued a similar report in May 2017. Cancer Research continues to explore and prove the correlation. Think of alcohol as an "over the counter" drug that should be managed accordingly.

- Avoid excess *caffeine,* which can impair insulin reaction, causing a detectable rise in blood sugar levels. Studies show that approximately 2 - 2.5 cups per day may cause this effect. (As someone who is extremely caffeine sensitive, I laughed when I read this research. If I drank that much coffee each day, I would have to be peeled off the ceiling!)

With regard to digestion and nutrition, caffeine inhibits the absorption of some nutrients causing the urinary excretion of calcium, magnesium, potassium, iron, and trace minerals. While tea may be a better choice overall, many teas contain caffeine, but also have an ingredient called thiamin, which helps buffer the caffeine effects.

I include energy drinks in the category of beverages to avoid for this reason. Excess caffeine interferes with the body's ability to absorb calcium, which is necessary to lay down bone. This is important to keep in mind if there is a predisposition to osteoporosis, or for teenagers, since most of our bone density is formed between the ages of 12 and 18. Sadly, more and more kids are developing caffeine habits through the use of coffee and/or energy drinks. Marketing and production of these products has skyrocketed over the past five or more years.

Excess caffeine can also cause excess stomach acid, leading to heartburn and indigestion. It can act as a stimulant to the bowel, causing diarrhea. It can even work like a diuretic on the bladder, leading to dehydration or urinary dysfunction. Here we have yet another good reason for increasing hydration with non-caffeinated beverages, primarily water.

Finally, caffeine is a stimulant that binds to adenosine receptors in the brain. This can lead to a range of complex reactions, causing an increase in stimulation of the adrenal glands. This in turn can increase our vulnerability to a variety of health disorders related to inflammation, general fatigue, "adrenal exhaustion" or even chronic fatigue syndrome. Because it is a stimulant, it can trigger the SNS to release stress hormones, making digestion more difficult. Caffeine is another one of those non-prescriptive drugs that can have strong effects that vary in intensity from person to person.

There are other concerns to consider when discussing digestive health, although they may not be about food and beverage. For example:

- Cigarettes and other tobacco products. Along with other environmental toxins these have been proven to be harmful. None of these is good for us—not chewing tobacco, not cigars, not pipes. There are new doubts, too, about the safety of vaping.

- Aerosols and body and beauty products.

These can be ingested by inhalation or by absorption through the skin. (If drugs can be transmitted through drug patches, so can skin care products!)

One common preservative found in many body lotions is *paraben*, rated by the EWG as a moderate to high health hazard. Another is *sodium lauryl sulfate* (SLS), an abrasive ingredient used in many shampoos, soaps and toothpaste to promote lathering, and to assist in removing dirt.

SLS is a sneaky, ubiquitous ingredient that may have negative effects, especially if you have skin or mouth sensitivities or frequent canker sores. One good line of products to try that shuns sodium laurel sulfate is Kiss My Face.

- Be aware of *bisphenol A* (BPA). This is a chemical used in making food and drink containers such as plastic water bottles and dishes. It is also used in the lining of canned goods. From these products, BPA can leach into foods and beverages, especially those prepared at extreme temperatures.

  It is important to avoid heating foods in plastic containers in the microwave. As an aside, heating and cooking food in a microwave can diminish the nutritional value of the foods we eat by "radiating" food with extremely high temperatures.

Similarly, try to avoid drinking water from plastic bottles that do not say BPA-free, especially if they have been stored in extremely hot or cold environments. Often, water bottles are stored in the freezer or hot storage spaces which promote the leaking of toxins into the water or contents.

- When buying and eating foods that are stored in cans, look for "BPA-free" on the labels. Fortunately, many food packagers now make their goods without BPA and are happy to promote this fact on their labels.

- Be aware of non-stick cookware, with surface coatings that contain PFOAs or *perfluorooctanoic acids*. These can cook off into our food, or release gasses into either food or the air, especially if the pots or pans are heated to very high temperatures. Chipped or scratched non-stick cookware should be discarded. To avoid using them at all, it is better to invest in cast iron, stainless steel or ceramic coated cookware.

Let's Get to the Bottom of Things

Moving further down the digestive tract, let's look at how we can support our colon and promote a healthy gut.

A *microbiome* is defined as a "community of microorganisms," for example, fungi, bacteria and viruses, living either in or on our bodies. There can be up to 100 trillion in and/or on one person, especially in the gut. Microbiomes are a hot topic these days in medical research, which is uncovering more and more connections between these organisms and illness, inflammation, disease and wellness.

Balancing one's microbiome goes beyond gut health. Our microbiome has a direct correlation to how well we absorb nutrients, how well our immune system works, the health of our brain, interaction with hormones and much more. Eighty percent of our immune system is located in our gut, and the digestive system is the second largest part of our neurological system. It is often referred to as our "second brain" and is known as the enteric nervous system.

To best promote a healthy balance of gut bacteria, consider the following guidelines:

- Avoid excess sugar and red meat. Bad bacteria love sugar and animal products.

Eat these minimally in order to keep the unhealthy organisms from proliferating. Too much bad bacteria in the colon can also produce excess gas by reacting with certain foods.

- Do not take antibiotics unless absolutely necessary. These medicines can kill good as well as bad bacteria.

- Limit the use of ibuprofen, which can erode the lining of the digestive tract, leading to ulcers and inhibiting the barrier needed to keep nutrients in and toxins out.

- Capitalize on good gut bacteria. Feed and replenish with fermented foods, acidophilus and probiotics.

- Include both *probiotics* (the healthy gut bacteria) and *prebiotics* (the fibrous "fertilizer" that promotes the growth of probiotics) in our diet.

- Eat onions and garlic. These are both antimicrobial foods that kill bad bacteria. They also contain *inulin,* which feeds the healthy flora in our gut, making them a prebiotic. These can be added to salads, or to any number of main dishes. Garlic is best eaten raw, or cooked slightly by adding it to the end of a sauté. If overcooked, garlic loses its nutritional value.

- Add fermented foods such as pickled ginger, sauerkraut and beets or homemade pickles to the diet. Ferment foods by brining with salt not vinegar. Vinegar does not have the full fermented or enzyme value that true fermentation using salt and time does. These products can also be purchased at a health food store, where they are usually kept in the refrigerated section.

  Be advised that the pickles we know from the grocery store shelf are made with vinegar and are often processed at high heat. This processing kills the byproducts needed in the natural lacto-fermentation process, resulting in a loss of their true value. Fermented foods are most effective in aiding digestion if they are eaten either during or at the end of a meal.

  A simple quick and easy way to brine vegetables is to mix 1½ tablespoons of sea salt and one quart of filtered or non-chlorinated water in a glass container. Cap the jar and shake it well to dissolve the salt. Add spices as desired (garlic, dill, horseradish, etc.). Wash several small, organic vegetables like cucumbers, cabbage, beets, onions, asparagus or any other desired vegetables. Pierce each with a fork several times, to allow for absorption of the brine. Pack the vegetables in the jar and cover with brine mixture. Cover the jar and let it sit in a warm area out of direct sunlight for three days. Then move to a dark, cool area for two to six weeks. Taste test the vegetables at various intervals while they are fermenting and adjust the time and add spices as desired. Refrigerate after opening.

- Try some home brewed beers—they have fermented qualities that commercial beers do not. The latter are usually made with preservatives and are processed at high temperatures that kill healthy bacteria.

- Eat yogurt, if dairy agrees with you. It is a great food known for its probiotics. It often contains acidophilus which is a particular strain or type of probiotic. But read the label and watch for excess added sugar. Greek yogurts are a best buy since they are higher in protein than regular yogurt. Kefir is another dairy-type product that contains healthy pre- and probiotics. Kefir contains less lactose than most dairy products due to the lactic acid content. This helps break down lactose via fermentation, but it still may not be a good choice for those who are either casein sensitive or vegan.

- Give kombucha a try. It is a quality probiotic drink that can be purchased in most health food stores and fermentories, or created at home. It is made from black or green tea and utilizes a process of further colonizing or fermenting bacteria and yeast from raw honey or cane sugar. This beverage is gaining in popularity but again, buyers need to watch out for excess added sugar. Pasteurization of kombucha is controversial, as it kills the good bacteria due to the high temperatures used during the process. If you prefer not to drink alcohol, be aware that kombucha does contain a small amount which is created during fermentation. My husband and I often think of kombucha as a soda alternative and a great "mocktail" when placed in fun glassware.

- Take a high quality probiotic supplement if it has been prescribed properly by a physician. Unless noted on the label, most probiotics need to be stored in the refrigerator to help preserve the bacteria. Good gut bacteria can help fight the bad bacteria, balancing the flora in your digestive tract. They are best taken with a meal to keep the digestive juices from destroying them before they reach the large intestine.

Without actually testing a stool sample to determine the exact makeup of gut flora, it is difficult to tell whether a probiotic supplement is necessary and what type. They can most definitely be useful, especially following a course of antibiotics where both good and bad bacteria get eliminated. Natural probiotics from our food rather than pills is most desirable as they are more easily absorbed from food-based sources but can be very helpful when prescribed by a trained medical professional.

Finally, no discussion of the lower end of the digestive tract would be complete without covering the actual process of defecation. Optimal bowel movements occur in a relaxed manner. The most important thing to remember about taking care of your bowel is to take care of business as soon as you feel the urge. Do not allow feces to sit in the end stages of the digestive system for extended periods of time. This waste product needs to be eliminated promptly. The longer stool sits in the bowels, the more it is apt to lose hydration and become compacted, which leads to constipation. Some people are very particular around toileting. They "hold" their bowels intentionally for hours (or days) until they can relieve themselves in the privacy and cleanliness of their own bathroom. While understandable, this habit can cause significant digestive and elimination issues.

Something else to keep in mind is actual body positioning for success. When seated on the toilet for a bowel movement, knees should be at the same level or higher than hips. If necessary, place a step stool under the feet. (Fans of TV's "Shark Tank" may be familiar with the Squatty Potty, a stool-like product that optimizes this proper poop posture.)

When I was a child my grandmother used to ask, "Did you go movie today?" At first I wasn't quite sure what she meant, but I knew the correct answer was "yes." Eventually, we figured it out and came to understand why this was important. (Grammy always did know best, even when it came to digestion and elimination.)

Know Your Body's Limits

When it comes to having a healthy digestive tract, being aware of our personal food allergies and sensitivities is critical. Knowing your body's tolerance for certain sometimes troublesome substances can be very helpful to aid digestion and the absorption of nutrients. Some foods can cause a wide range of sensitivity and allergic reactions. Even small amounts of certain foods, such as peanuts or shellfish, can lead to an extreme reaction or even death. Similarly, someone with celiac disease could have strong ill effects as a result of their gluten intolerance. Other people may respond to certain foods with mild symptoms that may worsen from a cumulative effect.

We often depend on medical testing to confirm allergies, but many of these sensitivities are not easily identified. There are tests for IgE versus IgG antibodies in the blood. IgG is a marker for a food sensitivity where the IgE is a marker for an allergy. Although I have no known allergies, I have experienced mild but notable symptoms of an allergic reaction that have certainly impacted my health and well-being, and not in a good way! Most of these reactions occur when I have eaten a troublesome food in excess or too frequently. I call this the cumulative effect. Through my naturopathic doctor, we have noted IgG's for certain food sensitivities like casein.

Some of the signs and symptoms that I have experienced over the years have included pounding headaches; red or watery eyes; eyelid styes; a stuffy nose; irritability and fatigue; extreme hunger; food cravings; muscle aches; canker sores and cold sores; rashes and acne; sleeplessness; swelling of my hands or feet and changes in my bowel or bladder patterns. Thankfully, with the help of my naturopathic doctor I have been able to identify and manage certain foods that are the most likely culprits. I have either begun eating less of these, eaten them less often, or eliminated them entirely from my diet.

If a food sensitivity or intolerance is suspected, the help of a doctor or physician recommended professional may be beneficial. An elimination diet may be recommended. I think of this as doing a personal study or science experiment. This can be done by eliminating certain foods or ingredients from the diet for two or more weeks and then reassessing the considered status or condition. After the set time, the questionable food is gradually reintroduced to see if a negative reaction occurs. It may be most helpful to try this with the guidance of an experienced professional.

Dairy, gluten (found in wheat, rye and barley) and sugar are three foods that frequently cause inflammation and irritation to the digestive tract. Different people have different tolerances or sensitivities to each of these, and they are not necessarily "bad" foods. They may be problematic temporarily if the gut is in a state of *dysbiosis* (microbial imbalance). Actually these foods may be able to be eaten later, in moderation, after symptoms have subsided and the gut has had a chance to heal.

Dairy products can cause an allergic or sensitivity type reaction for different reasons. Some people are adversely affected by the lactose or casein in dairy products. These can impact a number of bodily structures including the skin, or the digestive or the respiratory systems. People with asthma have been shown to improve with dairy elimination. My personal experience was with the cumulative effect of dairy on sinus infections. With an elimination diet, I was able to clear up my issue and am now able to eat dairy in moderation.

Dairy intolerance may not always be detectable by allergy testing, but can still cause trouble in the gut. We do not always need a medical diagnosis, positive allergy test result, or a medical professional to tell us to stop eating something. Maybe we have had allergy testing that came out negative but we know we do not feel well when we eat certain foods. By listening to our bodies and avoiding possible food irritants, we can manage a myriad of subtle irritating symptoms. We all need to learn to *trust our gut*!

If we find that we are more gassy or bloated, we can try eliminating certain sugary or starchy foods. Certain sugars and starches are not as easily digested and can cause gas. Lactose, which is a naturally occurring sugar found in milk and other dairy products, may be one of these. Try eliminating foods with lactose and see if symptoms improve. Similarly, gas and bloat may diminish by eliminating certain starchy foods such as potatoes, beans or cabbage.

Incompletely digested foods that reach the colon can react with gut bacteria to form even more gas, leading to bloating and gastrointestinal discomfort. This could be the result of a gluten sensitivity for some people. At other times, the symptom may not be due to an actual food sensitivity, but instead to incomplete chewing way back at the beginning of the digestive tract. Partially digested food is a common irritant to the colon so it's important to heed our earlier suggestion to chew every bite until it is quite soft.

Excess fiber in the diet is another known irritant to the colon. The undigested fiber can react with bacteria to cause distress. Varying the amount or type of fiber may be helpful until the right amount is determined. When eating high-fiber foods such as grains, remember to cook them well and chew them thoroughly. Beans and grains can also be soaked overnight or for a few hours before cooking to make them more digestible. A small piece of seaweed when cooking beans and grains can also be an aid. When eating canned bean, rinsing them well may be helpful in eliminating gaseous properties. Changing the type of fiber you eat is another idea. For example, slow-cooked oatmeal and quinoa are quite easy to digest if cooked appropriately.

Nightshade vegetables—tomatoes, potatoes, peppers, eggplant—is another food group that can cause bad reactions in some people. Studies have shown increased inflammation and exacerbating symptoms causing increased joint pain in some people after ingesting these foods. Most susceptible are those who have arthritis, especially rheumatoid arthritis (RA). Doing an experimental elimination diet of at least two weeks is well worth a try if body aches exist and a curious correlation around food, particularly the nightshade family, is suspected.

And Do Not Forget ...

When it comes to digestive health and wellness, I can not stress enough the importance and value of the following guidelines:

- Look to whole, natural foods for most nutrients and micronutrients, not pills and supplements.

- Eat plants from gardens, not food from manufacturing plants.

- Buy food that is minimally processed and with the fewest ingredients—mostly items that do not come in boxes or packages.

- Cook and eat most meals at home. Restaurant food is often over processed, too salty, and loaded with fat.

- Make home cooking fun and easy. Use quality knives, utensils, pots and pans.

- Read food labels! Look for hidden sugars, trans fats and added sodium.

- Relax, breathe. Get up early enough and do not start the day in a rush.

- Eat a proper breakfast. It sets you up for a good day.

- Drink 6-8 cups a day of clear, non-caffeinated, non-sugar fluids.

- Eat at regular times, as much as every three to five hours to prevent crashing and reaching for unhealthy boosters like caffeine or sugar.

- Avoid grazing. Give the digestive system time to recover between just two or three quality meals and a couple healthy snacks.

- Finally, stop eating at least three hours before bedtime.

With regard to ending the day, preparing for sleep, and what happens at night, Dr. Dale E. Bredeson explains in his book *The End of Alzheimer's* that allowing the digestive tract time to rest for three hours before bed actually facilitates the natural release of melatonin and promotes good quality sleep. Our best detoxing occurs in the hours leading up to bedtime, sleep time and in the early hours of the day.

Ideally, we should stop eating three hours before bed and abstain from eating for 12 or more hours from the last meal in the evening to the next meal in the morning. For example, if we complete dinner by 7 p.m. we should not eat again until breakfast the next morning at 7 a.m. With inflammation related to an existing illness, the body may actually need more time to detoxify, possibly up to 14 hours.

I like to think of this cleansing time as being similar to the time when the janitor or cleaning service goes into a school or business after hours and cleans up when nobody is in the building. Eating too close to bed can increase inflammation and change the body's focus for the evening. Spacing food properly is an easy way to promote quality sleep, wellness, healing, and weight loss. I recommend following Dr. Bredesen's "12/3 Theory" for a trial period of two to four weeks and then reassessing.

As always, with medical concerns, consult with the primary care physician or other trained health care professional.

For further reference

Dr. Joel Furman (www.drfurman.com)
Dr. Mark Hyman (www.drhyman.com)
Institute of Functional Medicine (www.ifm.org)
Institute of Integrated Nutrition (www.integrativenutrition.com)
Dr. Andrew Weil (www.drweil.com)

Chapter 6: Sleep and Healthy Sleep Habits

Why is sleep important?

Sleep is when growth and optimal healing and regeneration occurs. It is also the primary time that our detoxification systems work, which is part of healing and eliminating inflammation and toxins that have accumulated during the day. A lack of sleep can increase inflammation in the body, leading to illness and disease. If frequent fatigue is an issue with a client, I invite a review of sleep habits.

Does our personal sleep world need some attention? Note how much growing babies sleep —a lot. Notice how we are so much more tired when we are sick, diseased or in the process of healing or recovering from an injury or surgery.

Researchers have examined the scientific literature and discovered a link between lack of sleep and inflammation, just one of the identified side effects of sleep deprivation. Based on a review of 72 reports, which involved more than 50,000 participants from population-based and clinical studies, they concluded that getting too little or too much sleep resulted in increased inflammation levels.

"It is important to highlight that both too much and too little sleep appear to be associated with inflammation, a process that contributes to depression as well as many medical illnesses," said Dr. John Krystal, editor of *Biological Psychiatry*. Improved sleep can improve the natural immune response to fight illness and disease.

Sleep disturbances, such as waking up several times throughout the night or being unable to fall asleep (both in the category of insomnia), are examples of poor sleep. Getting less than, or more than, 7-8 hours of sleep per night has been shown to result in increased levels of inflammatory markers in the blood, like cytokines, C-reactive protein (CRP) and interleukin-6 (IL-6).

With inadequate sleep, inflammatory proteins and blood sugar levels rise in response to lower levels of insulin being released throughout the night. Decreased sleep resembles insulin resistance, causing an increase in glucose contributing to inflammation and diabetes.

Leptin, the satiety hormone, is significantly reduced when we are sleep deprived. Since leptin plays an important role in appetite control and metabolism, having low levels of this hormone results in hunger not being naturally suppressed. Therefore, appetite and cravings increase when our sleep is compromised. This too can lead to illness and obesity.

Melatonin is a hormone directly affecting our sleep and will be addressed in this section. A number of elements can improve or impede its release and function.

Let's review some healthy sleep habits.

Food and Drink

- Avoid eating within three hours of bedtime. As previously mentioned, Dr. Bredeson, a neurodegenerative disease expert and professor at UCLA, states that the natural release of melatonin is interrupted by the spike in insulin from digestion caused by eating too close to bedtime. Try to eat dinner early enough to allow adequate time for digestion before sleep.

- Take note of foods that disturb personal sleep habits and avoid them or limit eating them to earlier in the day. A variety of spicy or garlicky foods may be among the culprits. Be aware of the influences of foods and how they impact sleep patterns. If connections are unclear, try reflecting on daily intake by keeping a food journal that also includes the quality of sleep. Track data such as actual bedtime, how many hours of sleep occur, the number of times awakened and the cause, if known (for example, the need to urinate), and the time of awakening in the morning.

- Avoid stimulants such as caffeine, nicotine, and alcohol too close to bedtime. While alcohol is well known to speed the onset of sleep, it disrupts sleep later in the cycle as the body begins to metabolize it, causing arousal. I think of this as a rebound effect. Alcohol is a relaxant with a delayed stimulant affect. Remember that chocolate has caffeine and can also interfere with proper sleep.

- Avoid caffeine after lunch or later in the day. People usually know how caffeine effects them and how late in the day they can ingest it without disturbing their sleep. Everyone is different. Be honest with personal experience. If sleep is not ideal but caffeine effects are unclear, do a personal study. Try avoiding caffeine after midday for a week and see if sleep patterns change. Personally, I have to avoid caffeine after 3 p.m. but my husband is less sensitive to caffeine and is able to drink coffee before going to bed.

- Avoid continuous use of caffeine to artificially boost energy levels or to stay awake. Not only will this disturb the quality of sleep, it also could promote illness. The stimulant taxes the immune system by making it perform in overdrive and by stressing the adrenals. Caffeine adds to the release of cortisol, causing a stress reaction which can exaggerate the sympathetic nervous system. This can both interfere with sleep and cause anxiety.

- Avoid fluids within two hours of bedtime. If a middle of the night bathroom visit is necessary, make sure there is a clear, safe and dimly lit path for minimal sleep disturbance. Avoid middle of the night conversations. Gently and quietly go to and from the bathroom, return to bed softly and float back into deep rest with relaxing breaths.

Activities and Exercise

- Avoid brain stimulating activities before going to bed or while in bed. Do not take electronic tablets, computers or smart phones into the bedroom!

- Avoid stressful conversations or problem solving, intense books or reading materials, writing serious matters, watching stressful TV, participating in serious phone conversations, or even using a computer or cell phone within an hour before bed.

- Avoid exercising within two hours of bedtime. Physical activity can promote good sleep when performed at the right time of day. Vigorous exercise is best done in the morning or late afternoon. However, a relaxing exercise, such as yoga, can be helpful before bed to help initiate a restful night's sleep.

Medications

- Avoid sleeping pills if possible. Most doctors do not prescribe sleep medication for periods longer than three weeks. They can be very addictive and have multiple side effects, one actually being sleep interference. Try natural methods talked about here or discuss natural alternatives with your doctor, such as melatonin. Even long-term use of over-the-counter melatonin can disrupt the body's natural production and release of melatonin itself. If current sleep medications are being taken, consult with the concerning doctor and discuss weaning from it by implementing some of the healthy sleep habits discussed here. Especially important—do not drink alcohol while taking sleeping pills.

- Remember that "artificial sleep aids give artificial sleep." Sleep cycles are actually altered and often incomplete with prescription sleep medication. Try to manage sleep conservatively before taking sleep aids. If medication becomes necessary, try the lowest doses for a short period of time. Review other options with qualified sleep specialists and holistic health practitioners. Acupuncturists and herbalists can also be helpful.

Taming the Mind

- If hours are passing, all methods of relaxation have been tried and sleep just is not happening and stress levels are rising, it is best to simply get up and do something relaxing and peaceful. This will look different for different people. Guided meditation, reading a peaceful, calm book or journaling may be a few options.

- Try to eliminate or manage worrisome events and factors. Work on stress management. If stress interferes with sleep, explore the problem with your primary care doctor or request a referral to a qualified therapist. A talk therapist or counselor may be helpful in managing stress and resolving issues. Do not put off dealing with lasting issues that may be interfering with sleep and wellness. Try to find a time during the day to process worries and concerns, but not at bedtime. Bed is a place to rest, not a place to worry. Try to avoid emotionally upsetting conversations and activities before trying to go to sleep. Do not dwell on or bring problems to bed. Leave them outside the door.

- Practice positive thoughts and focus on gratitude at bedtime. This is the perfect time to reflect on the simple joys from the day and things we are grateful for. Create boundaries around the sleep space. Make it sacred. Agree to declare the bedroom a positive place.

- Do not go to bed if there is not even a hint of sleepiness.

- Begin rituals that promote relaxation each night before bed. Regular meditation and calming rituals can also help balance the neurotransmitters that directly affect the release of melatonin. Cortisol is a common stimulant that coincides with adrenaline and with excess stress it can rise to levels that may be unhealthy. If these levels are elevated at bedtime, they can have an inverse relation with melatonin and negatively affect sleep. Serotonin is another neurotransmitter. It is produced in the gut and aids relaxation. If serotonin levels are out of balance or low, we can become more stimulated and less able to relax. If our gut is in dysbiosis, serotonin production and uptake can be altered, yet another reason to promote a healthy diet and good digestion.

- Calming activities may aid in balancing the autonomic nervous system (ANS), leading to relaxation in general and to sleep preparation specifically. These practices may include such things as taking a warm bath, enjoying a light snack, listening to soft music, or doing some light reading. Reading or listening to a calming bedtime story also works for some people. There are a number of relaxation tools that can be downloaded from the Internet or accessed as a cell phone app or even viewed on YouTube. Focused breathing and other meditation techniques may also be helpful. Balancing the ANS as mentioned throughout this book can be extremely helpful with all aspects of health.

Schedule

Kenneth Wright, an integrative physiology professor at the University of Colorado Boulder, has researched the connection between sleep and exposure to the outdoors. He found that melatonin levels rise and fall naturally with sunset and sunrise if we are exposed to daylight and fresh air. His first study was done over a six-week period, then repeated over a two-day period. Both studies showed an immediate reset of the body's natural melatonin levels with increased exposure to outdoor natural light. In other words, we need to think about *when* we sleep as much as about how long we sleep. A few suggestions:

- Ensure adequate exposure to natural light and fresh air during the day. Light exposure helps maintain a healthy sleep-wake cycle. Try to get some natural daylight and outdoor time regularly. Go for a walk or sit outside often. If outdoor time is not a frequent option, then at the very least, spend time by an open window. At home or work, open shades and be exposed to daylight whenever possible. Fresh air and outdoor time can also help acclimate us to our environment, especially in the cold weather. Bundle up and go for a walk, even in the cold. This can help us become more tolerant of the cold season and sleep better. It may also lead to an improved mood and more energy.

- Avoid exposure to blue light within two hours of bedtime. Blue light is best known to exist in electronics and energy efficient light bulbs. During the day, blue light can be helpful to alertness, but near bedtime it can decrease the natural release of melatonin. Filtering glasses or screens on phones and computers can be used to help decrease unnecessary exposure.

- Keep a regular schedule throughout the day so the body can develop healthy habits and routines. Supporting the body's circadian rhythms can be helpful in promoting healthy sleep. Maintain regular times for meals, medications, chores, and other activities. This will help keep the inner body clock running smoothly.

- Practice regular bedtimes and morning risings no matter what your age. Try to maintain a regular sleep cycle throughout the week. Avoid multiple days of short sleep during the week followed by days of long sleep nights on the weekend. Many people develop this schedule for workdays and weekends. As a rule, go to bed at the same time every night and get up at the same time every day, even on weekends and holidays. It is important that we not give all of our valuable time to our employer or even our family or friends. Rise and shine, create some free time to do what we want or need to do to enhance our life and well-being. We think we deserve to "sleep in," but honestly, we truly deserve healthy sleep cycles and wellness. Challenge this old mindset and take a little extra time in the morning to start the day fresh.

- Get a full night's sleep on a regular basis. Get enough sleep to feel well-rested nearly every day. An average of eight hours is optimal and recommended by sleep experts. Longer sleep is required to enter deep sleep and dream cycles to get full benefits.

- Avoid taking naps late in the day. If naps are needed, try to keep them short, ideally to less than one hour. Especially avoid naps after 3 p.m. as this can disturb the normal pattern of sleep and wakefulness.

- Avoid falling asleep on the couch before bed. Couch sleeping before bed makes it more difficult to fall asleep at bedtime and disturbs the sleep cycle. If sleep sneaks into the living room chair or couch, go to bed. If it is too early for bed, but too late for a nap, get up and do a wakeful activity or project. Try a stimulating cold glass of water or a few pushups or jumping jacks to awaken the system and buy more time before the proper bedtime.

- Keep your beds sacred for sleep and intimacy, and create a mood and environment that supports this. Leave everything else outside the bedroom.

- Put a healthy plant in the bedroom. This is good *feng shui*, as a plant absorbs negative energy, promotes quality air exchange and acts as a natural air purifier. The peace lily is one of the top ranked house plants and my favorite for this use. It is an easy plant to maintain and is pleasing to the eye with an occasional bloom. Lavender, jasmine, aloe and spider plants are also conducive to a healthy bedroom atmosphere, but trust personal instincts to choose the right plant. Any plant that feels calming and pleasing will promote good sleep.

- Make sure that the sleep environment is pleasant and relaxing. A comfortable bed, a comfortable room temperature—not too hot, not too cold, not too bright. Be Goldilocks and find the bed that's "just right."

- Make bed and the bedroom pleasant with relaxing colors. Choose sheets and blankets that breathe. Cotton, down or down alternatives that are healthy with natural fibers are great options. Include comfortable pillows that fit your personal style and extra pillows for propping, proper alignment and helpful body support.

- Promote a relaxing environment with essential oils like lavender or vanilla. Put a few drops on a pillow or on a cloth next to the bed, or invest in a small diffuser. Lavender soap or lotion used before bed also can be very soothing. Choose a favorite that is personally calming.

- Maintain a dark sleeping space to assist the natural release of melatonin. Melatonin is sensitive to light and can be negatively affected by small amounts of light in the bedroom during sleeping hours. Room darkening shades can be very helpful if light leaks in through bedroom windows. I like our small bare window that allows just enough light in in the morning so I can awaken naturally.

In closing, I think sleep atmosphere was best described by Dr. Michael J. Thorpy, MD, Director of the Sleep-Wake Disorders Center at the University of Maryland Medical Center when he said, "Make your bedroom quiet, dark, and a little bit cool. An easy way to remember this: it should remind you of a cave. While this may not sound romantic, it seems to work for bats. Bats are champion sleepers. They get about 16 hours of sleep each day. Maybe it's because they sleep in dark, cool caves."

Rest Well, Be Well!

As I have said before, it is important to "start where you are." Make small doable changes or take small steps toward sleep goals. Be kind with self compassion. Practice 90:10. Avoid extremes and rigidity when possible. Develop lifestyle habits, not unsustainable binge changes.

If sleep doesn't improve with conservative measures, a more thorough consult may be necessary with a primary doctor, functional medicine practitioner or sleep specialist. There may be underlying health issues, possible medications that are interfering with sleep, or hormonal influences or an imbalance that needs attention.

Sources for Sleep Information

Irwin MR, Olmstead R, Carroll JE. "Sleep Disturbance, Sleep Duration, and Inflammation: A Systematic Review and Meta-Analysis of Cohort Studies and Experimental Sleep Deprivation." *Biological Psychiatry.* 2016.

Harvard Health Letter. "Blue Has a Dark Side," May, 2012. Updated December 30, 2017.

<u>Chapter 7: Detoxification</u>

Minimizing or eliminating toxins in the body is critical for a healthy lifestyle. As we have seen, one way to "keep it clean" is by eating a wholesome diet. But even the "cleanest" lifestyles still produce waste and interface with toxins. In order to minimize our toxic load, it is important to optimally process and eliminate toxins and waste products from the body. These harmful substances may be in our food or beverages, or our environment. Some are obvious, yet many exist without us ever knowing about them. With this in mind, it is still essential to try to manage these elements as best as possible.

Our bodies are naturally quite smart and are designed to manage commonly occurring toxins and waste products on their own. However, if we are exposed to an excess of these substances they can accumulate and lead to inflammation and illness. To improve upon the body's effectiveness in eliminating toxins, the goal here is to both support and facilitate the body's natural processes of elimination by adopting a few extra healthy behaviors.

In addition to the healthy practices regarding areas already addressed—sleep, digestion, bowel and bladder function, liver support—consider the following ways to promote healthy and natural detoxification mechanisms.

Balancing the Autonomic Nervous System

When we spend too much time in the *fight or flight* part of this system or the sympathetic state, running in a constant state of overdrive, the body's natural mechanisms become rigid and ineffective. When the autonomic nervous system is in balance and is able to spend some time in the parasympathetic state, the body is better able to attend to rest, recovery, healing and detoxing. This happens in a primarily relaxed state, whether in the parasympathetic condition or in good quality sleep. So here is another vote for practices such as getting an adequate amount of consistent, high-grade sleep; meditating daily; practicing mindfulness; focusing on relaxation breathing; seeking out peaceful moments; and spending time in nature.

Promoting Circulation and Lymphatic Flow

First, before taking on any new activity or activities that affect circulation, it is important to be cleared by a medical professional. We want to be sure that our bodies are safe in relation to our personal medical concerns. That said, the lymphatic system is closely tied to the circulatory system. It is supported passively, by gravity, external stimuli, and our body's natural muscle pumping action. Ways to support it include:

Massage. The most familiar form is Swedish massage, which can influence circulation in the direction of the heart. By stimulating the skin it affects the nerves, muscles, glands and circulation. Lymphatic massage focuses on lighter strokes and zeroes in on those areas of the body that contain the greatest number of lymph nodes —the back side of the lower body, the fronts of the arms, the neck near the collar bones, the lower abdomen, the axilla (armpit area), and the groin.

Skin stimulation. In Chinese medicine, our skin is considered to be the third kidney and one of our largest organs. It can be influenced through a variety of techniques. One method is called *dry skin brushing*. Just as the name suggests, this involves using a dry cotton washcloth or a natural fiber sponge or brush directly on the skin.

Dry skin brushing is a common practice in Eastern and Ayuverdic medicine that has been prescribed for many years. In addition to promoting circulation, dry skin brushing also loosens dead skin cells to make it easier for the skin to breathe, and to allow sweat to be released through the pores more freely. Most brushing is done in small circular patterns with gentle pressure and in the direction of the heart to facilitate circulatory and lymphatic effects.

When brushing, it is important to avoid areas of the body where the skin may be irritated or frail. And, of course, open sores should not be brushed. It is also important to consult with a doctor if you have any condition which makes you unsure whether brushing is safe. Most times the practice is quite safe and helpful, and do not be surprised if you experience the added benefit of a more youthful appearance as a result of skin brushing.

Another way to stimulate the skin is with a *hot washcloth rub*. This is an additional Eastern medicine technique popular among practitioners of alternative medicine. This type of rub is best done using a sink or basin of hot water and a natural cotton washcloth. The primary areas to rub are just above the collar bones, around the armpits, along the abdomen, and on the inner thigh or groin area. A rub can also cover the entire body, bringing benefits from top to bottom, or from distal limbs toward the central body or heart region.

The washcloth should be rinsed and wrung out frequently (no need to change the water) to maintain the heat effects. Practitioners often suggest completing a hot washcloth rub either before or after a shower, but you can also give yourself a rub during a shower if that is easier. Most often people do quick rinse showers without using a washcloth or actually scrubbing the skin.

A washcloth rub is an easy addition to one's daily hygiene and a beneficial aid in the removal of dead skin cells to promote deeper health.

Exercise

Movement has many detoxification benefits that vary, based on the type of exercise performed, and aids in both blood and lymphatic circulation, bowel function, air exchange, sweating, skin cleansing and mentally de-stressing. (Remember! Medical clearance is essential before starting a new program of exercise.)

Different types of exercise include cardiovascular workouts, weight training, stretching, yoga, tai chi, Pilates, dance and basically any movement that gets one away from sitting! Interval training is a hot topic these days and continues to be studied for its multiple benefits, detoxing being one of them. During interval training (such as HIIT or high intensity interval training) one varies the expenditure of effort from high to medium to low and back again several times. This type of workout can be as simple as a 20-minute routine of biking, running or elliptical training that includes increasing the intensity for 30 to 60 seconds every three minutes. When clients have coupled HIIT with a cleaner diet, I have actually seen them eliminate cellulite, a visible sign of detoxing and an absolute bonus esthetically.

Yoga has become increasingly popular in recent years for its many health perks for both mind and body. For example, yoga fans claim inversion postures and twists (putting your feet up the wall or rotating your spine) are particularly effective for detoxing. Incorporating what is called a sun salutation—instructions are readily available on the Internet or through YouTube—into your day can provide multi-dimensional benefits, even if performed briefly.

Start where you are and add movement to your daily life. Seek instruction and classes to learn proper techniques and create accountability. Regular activity will aid overall wellness.

The lungs are another natural detox organ, eliminating toxins through exhalation. This process occurs daily without effort or even thinking about it, but it can be enhanced by exercising to cleanse the lungs of carbon dioxide and to allow for an increase in oxygen intake. This, in turn, enhances our blood quality, circulation and wellness. Given these benefits, some people have turned to dedicated and vigorous *breath work*. (Although I am not all that familiar with this practice, I wanted to mention it and encourage readers to learn more about it if it sounds intriguing or personally beneficial.)

A few more therapeutic ways to increase blood flow and help flush the lymphatic system include relaxing in a sauna or steam room; taking hot and cold contrast showers, baths or plunges; soaking in an Epsom salt bath or enjoying a similar foot soak; and simply swimming in the ocean.

There is limited research on these methods but they all are strong elements of Eastern medicine and I have used a variety of these in my physical therapy and massage practices. In more recent years I have learned about their actual detox effects and am very intrigued by their effectiveness. I am a big fan of contrast baths, especially for injured limbs and combined hot and cold pack treatments for various states of ailments. Frequently, I prescribe Epsom salt baths for athletes with sore muscles or those suffering from arthritis. What is especially good about these techniques is that they are drug-free and minimally invasive so with proper guidelines they are well worth a try. A simple warm bath or shower can be very relaxing while helping to balance the nervous system and set us up for detoxification, healing and wellness.

<u>**Conclusion**</u>

Now that we have covered the basics for how to improve our diet and lifestyle, some extra suggestions may be helpful for carrying out the desired alterations and modifications. (This makes me think of that popular quote from the Bible: *"The spirit is strong but the flesh is weak." [Matthew 26:41]).*

Oftentimes it is not as easy to make changes as we think. More often than not, we know what we need to do, but actually implementing change and doing what is best for us can be extremely challenging. Education is only part of the equation for improving our health. There are many forces working against us. Social pressures and expectations from friends and family, long lived habits and routines, emotions, desires, fatigue, stress and more can sabotage our best intentions.

What follows are some tips to aid us in our journey to improved wellness.

Adopt an accountability partner.

During my health coach training through the Institute of Integrated Nutrition, we frequently worked with accountability partners to help us accomplish our goals and complete certain tasks. This "partner" was someone to keep us on target and to provide encouragement.

We can ask a friend, coworker, colleague or family member to walk the journey with us. The goal or task may be different for each of us, but we agree to make a personal commitment to ourselves to adopt a behavior for a certain period of time and have regular check-ins to hold each other accountable. Having someone other than just ourselves can be helpful in carrying out the desired action items.

I have successfully utilized this concept on a number of occasions. Years ago, a neighbor friend and I applied this to house cleaning. We agreed to clean our homes room by room thoroughly one week at a time. The first week we were in the kitchen, the next week the living room and on and on until we made our way through the house. Each week we would check in, sometimes in person, other times by text, phone or email. This made our tasks more fun and assured focus and completion.

During the past couple years, I have utilized health and life coaches, editors and peers to accomplish the completion of this book. It was much easier to be accountable to an external being rather than to myself alone. Sharing this journey has been very helpful, fun and more assuring of success.

For example, maybe we can recruit our spouse or child to walk the Dr. Bredeson plan to improve sleep and detox with us. As you recall, this means eating our last meal three hours before bedtime and 12 hours before the first meal of the next day. But whatever the change you focus on, having a cohort can make the deed less daunting.

Keep it simple.

This basic concept has been cited multiple times throughout this book, but is worth another mention.

Set yourself up for success by implementing small steps. Maybe you are exercising sporadically and want to increase the frequency of your workouts.Try setting a goal of taking some moderate exercise twice a week for 20 minutes instead of vowing to go to the gym every day. As you succeed, it will be easier to up the ante bit by bit until you reach your ultimate goal.

Knowing that the desired amount of exercise suggested by the American Heart Association is 75 to 150 minutes per week at a moderate level of intensity may feel overwhelming if you are only performing 40 minutes a week, but if we move gradually in the right direction, it becomes easier to stay on task and not give up. Smaller more achievable goals are the focus.

Maybe it's more vegetables that we need. The American Heart Association suggests eating seven to eight or more servings of vegetables and fruits per day and this may also feel daunting if we are stuck in the SAD (Standard American Diet) of one or two per day. Simply increasing by one more vegetable or fruit per day for a week could be the place to start while gradually working toward a long-term realistic goal of five vegetables and two fruits per day.

It is more useful to break down your goal into steps and to stay positive, maintaining your focus on what *will* be done rather than on what will *not* be done. Make basic doable goals with positive action steps, for example, instead of saying "I will not eat junk food," try saying "just for today I am going to eat plants vs. plants (manufactured foods)." Or, instead of saying "I will not drink soda," set a goal of increasing your water intake each week until you can consume a third of your body weight in ounces each day. (That's 50 ounces if you weigh 150 pounds.)

Focusing on the positive is a great way to *crowd out* poor diet and lifestyle habits. For example, if we are drinking more water that leaves less room for soda or sugary drinks. Or if we are exercising more, we have less time to sit on the couch eating junk food snacks.

Practice Gratitude.

I sometimes think I have heard this phrase a million times but I still love it. Whether it be in our heads or on paper or in cyber space, it is a great idea to keep a gratitude journal. Every day in this journal we can make a note of what we are grateful for. What a great way to finish the day on a positive note and add to quality sleep and pleasant dreams. Creating a sense of success and fulfillment in our lives leads to more success and fulfillment. With the natural tendency to focus on our failings (and those of others), this may be a bit of work, but it offers great rewards.

Utilize personal character strengths.

According to the VIA (Values in Action) studies, one of the lowest rated character strengths is *self-regulation*. It is no wonder making diet and lifestyle changes is such a struggle.

In my Functional Medicine Health Coach training, we have explored a lot of positive psychology and motivational interviewing. Some of my favorite work has been done with the non-profit the VIA Institute on Character. The founder, Dr. Neal H. Mayerson, has been involved in the study of positive psychology in the social sciences since 1998. Along with colleagues Dr. Chris Peterson and Dr. Martin Seligman, Mayerson has researched and assessed positive personality traits, and the group has created a "scientifically validated survey" that allows people to do a free online test that ranks 24 strengths in order of high to low. These characteristics represent common and desirable behaviors we display regularly, but some we may not be fully aware of.

Knowing that self-regulation is not one of the easier traits to implement, it is helpful to know what other strengths we more naturally exhibit so we can capitalize on these for greater success in personal growth. The natural human tendency is to live in a negativity bias, focusing on the dark side of life. Bringing attention to the gifts we already have can significantly add to our wellness goals.

Some of the top ranked strengths are kindness, fairness, honesty, gratitude and judgment. Maybe we can imagine how pairing one of these with a healthy task could be beneficial. Applying our own personal skills can enhance success.

The VIA group has proven that when we practice our top strengths regularly, we are happier and more easily able to make positive changes in our lives.

One of my favorite tools for implementing personal growth changes to better our lives is through the application of some of the top strengths recognized in the free VIA survey. I

encourage everyone to go online
(www.viacharacter.org) to find your top strengths.
Knowing these and applying them can make
working toward personal growth more effective.
The website also offers great explanations and
tools to help implement the use of one's
strengths. It may also be helpful to work with a
certified health coach trained in positive
psychology to increase your success rate.

Be proactive.

In functional medicine coach training, we are
taught to explore the obstacles that may
challenge the new healthier behaviors. We are
taught to think ahead for troubleshooting.

For example, if you have a special occasion or a
vacation upcoming, give it some forethought.
Where will the barriers be? What is a realistic
goal or action step in that environment? What are
some ideas to implement? Is it a wedding?
Maybe we decide to simply join in the
champagne toast then abstain from alcohol and
drink seltzer water with lime or create a soda
juice, have one bite of cake but not a whole
piece, dance more and eat less, leave before the
band stops. Inform a friend or family member of
your plan and ask for support.

Find meaning and purpose in health goals.

Instead of simply living a healthy lifestyle because we know it is the right thing to do, make it personal and desirable and something you want to do. By having a vision for the future, we give our action items greater purpose.

For example, eating better, getting more exercise and improving our sleep can give us the energy to be active and play with our children or grandchildren. Eating more low starch vegetables and fruits along with lean proteins and quality fats to improve our blood work may mean we can decrease the need to take cholesterol or pre-diabetic medications. Maybe the goal could be about doing our part to prevent the repeat of a family disease or illness by breaking the cycle of unhealthy diet and lifestyle.

As a physical therapist, I have witnessed patients that vary in their home compliance. With advancing my training into health coaching and the study of positive psychology and motivational interviewing, it has been very intriguing to explore human behavior and how to enhance outcomes by applying some of these newly added skills. I have clearly learned the value of *less is more,* keeping it simple, and helping clients find meaning and purpose in their goals. Motivating people with authentic positivity and affirming feedback has also been validated as an effective approach for success. And, exploring barriers to performance and troubleshooting backup plans has become an added bonus.

Be a science experiment.

Try doing a trial for two weeks. Make a healthy diet or lifestyle change, then see what happens. Notice if you have more energy, improved sleep, less congestion, decreased pain, improved bowel health or any simple or even major change for the better. Just notice, be aware. Repeat and tweak the experiment as needed for optimal results.

Listen to your barometer.

We all have internal voices that talk to us if we listen. Our bodies are wise and try to message us about our interface with, and the effects of diet and lifestyles. Is it headaches, fatigue, sleep disturbances, irritability, skin changes, body aches or digestive issues that are the problem? Take mental notes of consistent patterns that occur. For me it is sinus congestion that speaks the loudest and mostly in relation to dairy products.

Create a *personal prescription for wellness.*

Everyone has certain things they know make them feel well. I know I feel better, sleep better and perform better both mentally and physically when I incorporate certain habits into my daily routine. For me, some of these are getting regular exercise, drinking more water, not snacking after dinner, spending more time in nature, connecting with friends and family, cutting back on alcohol, and eating fewer refined wheat products, dairy products and sugar. When these are in balance I usually feel pretty sharp and wholesome, generally well overall. Be aware of what works *for you,* and start to create that mental or written note of what does it *for you.* Shoot for 90:10 and do these things most of the time, allowing for small amounts of imperfection.

Make it fun.

Like the proverb says, *"all work and no play makes Jack a dull boy."* Engage others to join you in shopping for, chopping and prepping for, and cooking healthy dishes. Bring a buddy to the farmers' market. Invite a friend to cook and share a meal. Invite someone to eat out with you and make it a game to see how healthy the meal can be from beginning to end, from your drink choices to your soup or salad to entrée etc.

And do not forget to have fun rewarding yourself for success by connecting with an old friend, going to a concert, buying a new outfit, taking a trip to the beach, going on a hike or engaging in a nature outing. Maybe go somewhere new you have been wanting to visit. Just remember to make the prize a healthy one. We would not want to sabotage all of our good work!

Shine your light, ask for help.

Finally, to all of my readers I say *good luck,* and invite you to contact me with your questions and feedback, to share stories of your progress toward living a healthier lifestyle, or for assistance in meeting your wellness goals.

Be well!

<u>Acknowledgements & Gratitude</u>

Institute of Integrated Nutrition (IIN)

Functional Medicine Coaching Academy (FMCA, part of the **Institute of Functional Medicine,** IFM)

Lisa Silverman and her Five Seasons Cooking School, for several years of seasonal classes, and for sharing her knowledge on vegan foods and the Chinese Five Elements theory. Also, for introducing me to great guest lecturers, experts such as Warren Kramer from the Kushi Institute and Jessica Porter, author of *The Hip Chick's Guide to Macrobiotics*.

Meg Wolff, for her early teachings on healthy eating and cooking with macrobiotics, and for authoring *Becoming Whole* and *A Life in Balance*.

Amy Rolnick, for making her wholesome cooking classes such fun, for chopping vegetables with a smile, and for teaching me how to roll sushi.

Dr. Sarah Ackerly, ND, to whom I am most grateful for helping me to change my way of thinking and for sending me on a holistic journey of exploring natural wellness. And for continuing to be by my side.

Dr. Margaret Schoeller, MD, for taking great care of me during my childbearing years with a very grounded integrated approach and referring me to my lifelong naturopath Dr. Sarah.

For **family** and **friends**, whose love and support along this wellness journey has meant so much, and for encouraging me in this book process.

For my many **patients** and **clients**, for entrusting me to support them in their personal wellness journeys. Whether it be for physical therapy, massage or health coaching, thank you!

For my proof-readers and their personal and professional interest and expertise. Thank you, **Virginia Weaver**.

Carrie Aube, for her professional photography.

Andrew Weil, for offering me my early understanding of the basics of a healthy diet and wellness, as well as the importance of the autonomic nervous system (ANS), proper breathing, mindfulness and meditation for optimal health.

And last but not least, my terrific editor **Christine Palmer**, who helped keep me on track over the last few years to accomplish this compilation of wellness to share.

<u>Resources</u>

Mark Hyman —www.drhyman.com (functional medicine and holistic and natural wellness practices)

EWG— www.ewg.org (environmental toxins)

Shawn Stevenson — www.shawnstevensonmodel.com (sleep)

Institute of Integrative Nutrition (IIN) — www.integrativenutrition.com

Institute of Functional Medicine (IFM) — www.ifm.org

Kris Carr — www.kriscarr.com (wellness enthusiast and cancer survivor, whose own journey is an amazing story)

Andrew Weil — www.drweil,com (natural wellness practices)

Deepak Chopra — www.chopra.com (meditation and wellness)

Theresa Freeman — www.theresafreeman.org

<u>About The Author</u>

Theresa and her husband, Paul, live in Falmouth Maine. During the two year period Theresa was writing her book, she was intimately involved in her husband's brain cancer journey. They are eternally grateful for today and that Paul is a thriving survivor.

Together, they enjoy spending time in nature, with friends and family, being active or hitting the road to see their boys. The couple have two sons in college, Ben at the University of Connecticut and Jack at Boston College.

Theresa studied Physical Therapy at Northeastern University followed by an orthopedic and sports fellowship through the UNC Chapel Hill and the American Sports Medicine Institute. Her more recent studies have been in health coaching through the Institute of Integrative Nutrition (IIN) and the Functional Medicine Coaching Academy (FMCA). She has a passion for learning and loves to share her knowledge.

Ever the passionate health and wellness detective, Theresa dedicates herself to collaborating with her clients to help them discover small, doable changes that can often make a big impact on their whole well-being.